PRIMARY PROGRESSIVE APHASIA

Logopenic Progressive Aphasia (LPA), Nonfluent-Agrammatic Variant Primary Progressive Aphasia (naPPA), & Semantic Variant Primary Progressive Aphasia (svPPA)

JERRY BELLER HEALTH RESEARCH INSTITUTE

Copyright © 2019 Jerry Beller
All rights reserved.
ISBN-13: 9781654427108

DEDICATION

To people living with Dementia and their loved ones.

CONTENTS

FOREWORD 1

    Who is the reading audience? 5

    Two Dementia Series 14

I. DEMENTIA 16

    Chapter 1: WHAT IS DEMENTIA? 17

    Chapter 2: WHAT ARE THE 19 PRIMARY DEMENTIAS? 21

    Chapter 3: WHO IS MOST LIKELY TO GET DEMENTIA? 23

    Chapter 4: DEMENTIA COSTS & PREVALENCE 40

II. 19 PRIMARY DEMENTIA TYPES 53

III. PRIMARY PROGRESSIVE APHASIA DEMENTIAS 56

    Chapter 5: WHAT IS PRIMARY PROGRESSIVE APHASIA (PPA)? 57

IV. PRIMARY PROGRESSIVE APHASIA DEMENTIA SYMPTOMS 73

    Chapter 6: PRIMARY PROGRESSIVE APHASIA (PPA) SYMPTOMS 74

    Chapter 7: LOGOPENIC PROGRESSIVE APHASIA (LPA) SYMPTOMS 75

    Chapter 8: NONFLUENT-AGRAMMATIC VARIANT PRIMARY PROGRESSIVE APHASIA (naPPA) SYMPTOMS 76

V. PRIMARY PROGRESSIVE APHASIA RELATED STAGES 80

    Chapter 9: EARLY STAGE PRIMARY PROGRESSIVE APHASIA (PPA) 81

    Chapter 10: MIDDLE STAGE PRIMARY PROGRESSIVE APHASIA (PPA) 85

Chapter 11: LATE STAGE PRIMARY PROGRESSIVE APHASIA (PPA) 87

VI. PRIMARY PROGRESSIVE APHASIA DEMENTIA RISK FACTORS 90

Chapter 12: PRIMARY PROGRESSIVE APHASIA (PPA) RISK FACTORS 91

VII. BONUS SECTION 105

Chapter 13: Starter To-do List for Somebody and Family once Diagnosed with Dementia. 106

Chapter 14: CARE TEAM 114

Chapter 15: LETTER TO CONGRESS 121

CONCLUSION 124

THANK YOU FOR READING 128

BELLER HEALTH BOOKS 129

Other Beller Health Books 132

ABOUT THE AUTHOR 133

ACKNOWLEDGMENTS

Thanks to the American Academy of Neurology, Atlanta Center for Medical Research, Alzheimer's Association, Alzheimer's Disease Center, Alzheimer's Disease Center of Northwestern University, Alzheimer's Foundation of America, American Academy of Neurology, Association for Frontotemporal Degeneration, Australia Neurological Research, CDC, Department of Health and Human Services, Duke University Medical Center, Emory Hospital, Harvard Medical School, Johns Hopkins Medicine, Mayo Clinic, National Aphasia Association, National Institute of Neurological Disorders and Strokes, National Library of Medicine, National Institute on Aging, National Institutes of Health, Prince of Wales Medical Research Institute, *PubMed*, Stanford Library School of Medicine, Stanford Medicine, UCSF Department of Neurology, UCSF Memory and Aging Center, University of Cambridge Neurology Unit, World Health Organization (WHO), *Journal of American Medical Association* (JAMA), and several other organizations that provided information used for this book. Thanks to everybody who assisted this book in a variety of important ways, and everybody at Beller Health Research Institute. To my editor, John Briggs, who helps me improve every book. To all sources and for the photos. Most of all, thanks to my wife, Nicola Beller

FOREWORD

Before diving into the book's subject matter, let's discuss two related Dementia series:

- *2020 Dementia Overview* series
- *2020 Dementia Types, Symptoms, Stages, & Risk Factors* series

2020 Dementia Overview series is an extension of the medical groundbreaking *19 Dementia Types, Symptoms, Stages, & Risk Factors* series, the first covering all primary dementia types.

After spending decades building an audience in other genres, including nutrition, circumstances turned the world upside down. Doctors diagnosed my mother with Alzheimer's. The same doctors soon diagnosed my father with cancer. A few months later, my father's favorite brother and my closest uncle died.

Three consecutive hard blows blew the world beyond recognition.

Tough and decent as they come, dad insisted on taking care of my mother while fighting brain cancer. My brothers and sister-in-law did their share, but Dad cared for my mother for a long time while they worked. Dad proved what a remarkable and great man he was down the stretch but finally succumbed to brain cancer.

My brothers and sister-in-law did their best to take care of mom, but it came at a price. Caregiving for a dementia patient is an indescribable horror I would not wish on my worst enemy.

You must watch somebody you love wilt away, little by little until dementia wipes away huge chunks of their personality.

Living away, my wife and I visited when possible. We saw how mom deteriorated, but also the effect caregiving had on my father and brothers. It was like watching a train wreck over and over, each time getting worse and helpless to prevent it.

Watching Alzheimer's takedown, my strong-willed mother and others bruised my soul. My writing shifted initially to learn about Alzheimer's, but the more learned, the more I cringed.

The cold hard facts rendered me speechless. Over 5.8 million Americans, and 44 million people worldwide, suffer Alzheimer's. No cure. Just a devastating and expensive slow march towards an agonizing end.

Not content to kill, Alzheimer's tortured Mom for years before killing her. It robbed her memory and damaged her brain, where she repeated herself in a continuous loop, each time thinking she was saying it the first time. As the disease advanced, the neurological disorder destroyed her mind and body.

Seeing dementia take down that tough old bird rattled me. While I could not bring back my mother, I dedicate my life to researching and writing about dementia 8-12 hours per day, six or seven days per week.

I tackled Alzheimer's to learn everything I could about the brute and determine how I and others might prevent it and other noncommunicable diseases. Having written on nutrition and advocated health in Washington, I already had a clue but determined to figure out how to prevent Alzheimer's. But I needed to know more, much more, about this terrorizing neurological disorder.

I learned Alzheimer's was just one of over one-hundred neurological disorders causing dementia. When I searched for a book covering the primary dementias, none existed. Instead, I turned to individual books and again found no books written on several of the most frequent dementias.

In what on the one hand seems like yesterday and the other a lifetime ago, I set out several years ago to write a dementia book covering the 15 most prevalent dementia types. The first to do that, I next wrote books covering each of the 15 most prevalent dementias.

In 2020, I expanded the book covering 15 dementias to 19 dementia types. I also released books on each of the 19 dementias. While proud of these medical firsts, I do not take myself too seriously.

As one of the dozens of scientists, neurologists, researchers, and writers who devote their lives to fighting the war against dementia, I remain humble. I appreciate the individual and combined accomplishments of everybody else in the field.

Nor should any of us get cocky knowing we're losing the war. If we win the war during my lifetime, I will celebrate with hundreds of people worldwide who helped defeat the great beast of our day.

My two-book series break medical ground, and I consider major achievements but remain two among hundreds of significant contributions to the dementia field by people around the globe.

The series provides patients and loved ones a great resource for dementias not covered as extensive as Alzheimer's and the more prevalent types.

By covering the 19 most prevalent dementias, doctors, nurses, and medical professionals benefit from a series covering neurological disorders causing 99% of dementia. The series helps primary care physicians, providers, and nurses who struggle to diagnose dementias with overlapping symptoms.

The series is an organic, evolving work, and each book receives major annual updates. As science uncovers information, we add important data in new editions. We also polish each edition.

We describe the writing goal in three ways:
1. Simplify the language and make it easier for nonscientists to comprehend.
2. Honor the science and facts.

3. Document science and include citations for doctors, nurses, medical researchers, students, and patients.

Our goal is to provide invaluable medical information for professionals, patients, loved ones, and caregivers.

I do not reinvent the wheel but accumulate the best research and teach our readers a better understanding of Alzheimer's and the other 18 primary dementia types.

Among the worst news is one of our loved ones has dementia. A killer disease with no cure frightens the bravest souls.

This medical condition destroys, not just the inflicted, but their loved ones. Besides the patient, nobody suffers more than voluntary caregivers. Watching a mother, father, brother, sister, wife, or husband suffering dementia brutalizes the soul.

I study dementia year around to write and release annual updates to honor people—including my mother—taken by Alzheimer's or one of the other primary dementias.

Modest book royalties are the only compensation, as I accept no money from corporations to promote their product. Nor do I have an ax to grind with anybody in the medical profession.

Having written 100 plus books over four decades, I am thankful to readers for collectively providing me a decent income. However, now in my sixties, I care little about riches and fame.

Who is the reading audience?

The audience falls into five categories.

Those Diagnosed with Dementia

If doctors diagnose you with dementia, my heart goes out to you. You're in for a long battle. Do yourself a favor and focus on slowing the disease and extending the quality of life. One word of caution, the books in this series speak to not only patients, but also families, doctors, students, nurses, and caregivers. Many of those diagnosed with dementia appreciate and benefit from the books, but some find some of the material too disturbing. I intend to write books exclusively for patients but must finish the work related to this series first. While there is not anything too shocking, I wrote the material for a wide audience, meaning I am not always speaking to patients specifically. I promise to personalize an edition for patients and loved ones after finishing this series. By shining a light on all 19 primary dementia types, I hope to help the medical community better distinguish and diagnose neurological disorders.

Loved Ones of Those Diagnosed

If doctors diagnose a loved one with dementia, he or she needs you more than ever. Depending on the type, dementia causes behavioral problems, memory issues, motor decline, and other psychological and physical disorders. The learning curve is steep and changes as one moves from one stage to the next. As with those with dementia, I warn families these books provide a technical overview, and the emphasis is not always on the emotional aspect. If you want to learn about dementias, this series is a great option. If you're looking more for emotional support, there are more appropriate books. I also plan to write a book specifically for families once fulfilling responsibilities for this series.

Medical Professionals

If you are a medical professional interested in studying the dementias, the series covers the dementias responsible for 99%

of dementia. While neurologists probably already know the 19 primary dementias, the books provide a quick overview and reference for primary care physicians, nurses, other medical professionals, and students. I also include citations so you can continue your investigation beyond the book's scope.

Volunteer & Professional Caregivers

If you are a dementia caregiver, you are also in for a long, difficult march. Dementia patients demand 24/7 care in later stages, requiring help to go to the bathroom, bathing, and other basic daily functions. While this series is not written solely for caregiving, caregivers benefit by gaining a better understanding of each dementia, their symptoms, and progression.

Anybody Wanting to Learn About A Disease That Strikes 1 Of 6 Americans, And 1 Of 3 Seniors

The series benefits anybody who wants to gain an intermediate understanding of the 19 dementias.

Series' First Lesson

Doctors, like teachers, are part of a sacred profession. **Nothing I say or write replaces your need for a competent doctor!** Nor does any criticism of the profession diminish my respect and admiration for the best.

I detest the worst teachers who fail students and society but love and respect the best. Society would crumble without the most devoted and competent teachers.

Similarly, I abhor incompetent, greedy doctors who fail patients and society, but love and respect the best.

The profession must weed out incompetent, uncaring, corrupt doctors, and medical personnel. Every profession has a percentage of bad apples, but within the medical profession, they are cancerous!

Nothing good I write about the medical profession includes incompetent, uncaring doctors, researchers, nurses, etc. And nothing bad I write targets the best.

The series criticizes the profession when deserved, but the

first lesson in this series: **Find a competent doctor!** If you have one, count your blessings. If not, find one.

Just as one can learn outside the classroom, we live in a blessed age where medical information is available for anybody on the internet. Such information serves us well, but do not—for a minute-think it replaces the need for a competent, devoted doctor.

The Wrong Doctors

Let me begin this section by saying I love and respect quality doctors, nurses, researchers, and medical professionals from the bottom of my heart and the fullness of my mind.

However, this section is not about what's right in the medical profession.

Glorified idiots, bad doctors are dangerous parasites who dishonor a noble profession. Smart enough to finish medical school, but greedy or flawed beyond redemption, they are like priests working for the devil. Among the worse members of society are doctors motivated by greed or limited by incompetence. Walking parasites!

The Wrong Doctors + Big Pharm + Big Insurance + Big Hospital = Expensive & Inadequate Health Care

Over the past few decades, Big pharmaceuticals, Big Insurance, and their political puppets appointed doctors sanctioned drug dealers. Entrusting the worse doctors with such powers produces little or no better results than assigning the task to a thug on the worst corner in America.

The worst doctors who hand out drugs like candy serve nobody's purpose but their own and Big Pharm.

Not an indictment of the entire profession, but unfortunately, Big Insurance dictates the typical office visit includes a quick examination and one or more prescriptions. The approach is not based on good science and runs counter to everything science teaches us.

What About Some Tough Love?

The one thing people today do not want is what we often need most, tough love. People want everything sugarcoated and easy.

The problem is most of the time; life is neither sweet nor easy.

What patients need much of the time is not an alleged "magic pill," but instead tough love. Doctors must learn nutrition and teach patients to eat healthier, exercise more, and get 7-8 hours of sleep per night. Like it or not, this is part of modern medicine. Showing up and passing out pills all day is not preventing Alzheimer's and other dementias, nor curing them.

Medical professionals must lead by example and embrace the science of nutrition, exercise, and sleep. If a healthy diet and exercise are the two cornerstones to health, the third is sleep.

The average person needs few or no drugs if they practice healthy habits.

Any doctor who does not vigorously advocate a balanced whole food diet, exercise most days of the week, and 7-8 hours' sleep per night neglects their duty and

Instead, too many doctors ignore the three cornerstones of health and are content to write their patients unnecessary and potentially dangerous prescriptions for the rest of their lives. 100% emphasis on treating symptoms with drugs, which often require more drugs to counter the side effects, is producing disastrous results. To be the best doctor, one must also emphasize prevention.

Failed Drug Trials

None of the drug trials have produced even one drug that cures Alzheimer's and other dementias. While science has failed to produce any effective dementia drugs, scientific studies prove we can do much by practicing healthy habits to slow or reduce our dementia risk.

The Medical Profession Must Think Outside the Box

The hopeless circle of failed drug trials demands we think outside the box or, as neurologist David Perlmutter advocates, expand the box. He and other neurologists deserve credit for recognizing medicine is failing the dementia war and rocking the boat of conventional wisdom. I must not agree with every point "maverick" neurologists like David Perlmutter, Dale Bredesen, and Deepak Chopra make to respect them for turning conventional wisdom on its head.

Conventional wisdom is losing the Alzheimer's and dementia war!

Not Anti-doctors or Anti-drugs

I am not anti-doctors or anti-drugs and do not understand those who insist neither are needed. I revere competent doctors who practice and advocate the three cornerstones of health. I also recognize the polio vaccine and many other drugs as nothing short of miraculous.

But, my love for what is right about the medical profession will not silence me about what is wrong. And, pretending drugs are the answer to defeating Alzheimer's or dementia is a colossal failure.

You cannot "**do no harm**" and write prescription drugs at the volume of the average doctor.

Choose A Doctor with The Same Care as You Do A Spouse

Find a competent, dedicated, caring, experienced, informed, ethical doctor who listens and respects your opinion, and writes prescriptions as a LAST RESORT.

Without the right doctor, you are at the mercy of a profit-oriented health system that seldom puts the patient's interests first, second, or third.

Nothing I say or write in these books or elsewhere means you should not see a doctor, stop taking your medication, or otherwise undermine the medical profession's ability to diagnose and treat any medical symptoms you might experience.

Find a good doctor you trust with your life and ask him or her pointed questions concerning your health and any treatment they recommend.

Outside the Bubble

I challenge the medical profession where necessary, just as I criticize Congress and the United States government for their mistakes or shortcomings. My brief career as a Congressional staffer taught me how difficult it is to maintain one's focus inside the bubble.

Seeing the big picture is no less challenging inside the medical bubble motivated by profit.

Profiteers fund too many studies to promote their product or discredit somebody else's. Blatant self-interests taint studies and confuse the public. Such contradictory studies confuse and make it impossible for the average person to understand which studies to believe.

I respect ethical, competent, dedicated, and hardworking nurses, doctors, and other medical personnel. As much as I criticize what is wrong within the profession, I cannot praise the majority of medical professionals often enough. Getting quality medical care when we need it is one of life's greatest blessings.

Nor do I object to medical-related businesses making a reasonable profit in return for needed medical supplies and services.

Nor should any competent and ethical medical professionals object to anybody challenging medical incompetence and profiteers.

Trust Thy Doctor

The right doctor does not discriminate between physical and mental diseases, so hold back nothing if you or a loved one exhibits symptoms.

If you lack the right doctor, find the right one. Outside you and the daily habits you establish, nobody is more important than your doctor for your health. You must be able to tell him or her medical information you might be reluctant to tell your closest confidant in life.

Remember, doctors too often misdiagnose dementia. Once the symptoms of these deadly dementias set in, you need to see your doctor, provide them with all the information about your problem, and help the specialists reach the correct diagnosis.

Because no tests exist for most dementias, doctors order tests and go through a process of elimination until reaching a diagnosis based on the symptoms you report. The more information you provide, the better the chance of a quick and accurate diagnosis.

Adopt healthy lifestyle choices to prevent dementia when possible, but the next best option is to diagnose it early, to confront it head-on, and take steps to slow the disease. Once dementia hits, it's often possible to postpone the advanced stages. If you've seen a loved one inflicted with dementia, you understand how precious a year, a month, a week, or day is once the storm aims at you or a loved one.

Prolonging life in late-stage dementia without a cure amounts to cruel and unusual punishment, but patients, families, and doctors must do everything possible to extend quality of life while possible.

Make certain you have a doctor who believes in prevention and natural cures, but also remember you need their expertise concerning the best that modern medicine offers.

Be Your Nurse!

If you have a loved one, be each other's nurse. If not, be your nurse.

It's more important than ever for you to monitor your blood pressure and make notes of health issues as they arise. We don't go to the doctor every time we develop a symptom or don't feel well, but it's important to keep a medical journal. Write an outline of the problems you experience between visits.

Too often, we march into the physician's office and don't provide a full or accurate representation of our problem. For instance, if you track your blood pressure, you can furnish a pattern rather than a onetime reading. You can also perhaps attribute pikes in your blood pressure to stress taking place in your life.

You should also track other symptoms. Providing thorough information helps doctors eliminate multiple diseases with similar symptoms. When you document all or most of the symptoms that have led to the visit, you provide a competent doctor a clearer picture to develop a hypothesis. These previous unrelated symptoms might help your physician make more sense of what prompted the appointment.

Otherwise, your physician might order the wrong tests or prescribe the wrong drugs. For issues of the brain, you can't be shy or embarrassed about providing your physician with a full portrayal of your problems and symptoms.

Although still stigmatized in some circles, mental illnesses are just as real, and the sufferers are no more the blame, than physical disorders. While we must do everything in our power to avoid or slow mental or physical maladies, the last thing we need to do is embarrass those who are already suffering.

Two Dementia Series

The laborious task to document the primary dementias began as a fifty-page Alzheimer's overview. Two editions later, the 50-page Alzheimer's book turned into 400 pages.

One of the first lessons taught Alzheimer's is only one of the hundreds of diseases responsible for dementia. With inadequate testing, similar symptoms, and other handicaps, the medical community often misdiagnoses the other dementias for Alzheimer's.

My focus broadened from Alzheimer's to a dozen dementias. The only way to make any sense of Alzheimer's or dementia was to study all the primary dementias.

I worked with several neurologists and researchers over the next couple of years and hit every medical library I could hit in person or available online.

After an extensive review, I wrote the first book covering

the 15 most prevalent dementia types, which provided the groundwork for two updated dementia series.

The associated *Dementia Types, Symptoms, Stages, & Risk Factors, series* expands the collection by adding amyotrophic lateral sclerosis (ALS), early-onset Alzheimer's disease, amyotrophic lateral sclerosis, corticobasal syndrome, and progressive supranuclear palsy.

Two Dementia Series

Not counting mixed dementia, there are nineteen primary dementia types, which two groundbreaking series covers.

Dementia Types, Symptoms, Stages, & Risk Factors series

1. *Dementia with Lewy Bodies*
2. *Parkinson's Disease Dementia*
3. Corticobasal Syndrome
4. Typical Alzheimer's Disease
5. *Posterior Cortical Atrophy*
6. *Down Syndrome with Alzheimer's*
7. *Limbic-predominant Age-related TDP-43 Encephalopathy (LATE)*
8. Early-onset Alzheimer's
9. *Behavioral Variant Frontotemporal Dementia*
10. Progressive Supranuclear Palsy
11. *Nonfluent Primary Progressive Aphasia*
12. Logopenic Progressive Aphasia
13. *Cortical Vascular Dementia*
14. *Binswanger Disease*
15. *Normal Pressure Hydrocephalus*
16. *Huntington's Disease*
17. *Korsakoff Syndrome*
18. *Creutzfeldt-Jakob Disease*
19. Amyotrophic Lateral Sclerosis

*Not a dementia type, but a combination, mixed dementia is the 20th category important in dementia discussions.

Any disease leading to associated symptoms is a dementia type. The series breaks medical ground by covering the dementias responsible for over 99% of dementia cases.

Dementia Overview Series

The second series focuses on all the primary dementia types or breaks them down as groups.

2020 Dementia Overview Series

1. Dementia Types, Symptoms, & Stages
2. *Lewy Body/Parkinsonism Dementias*
3. *Vascular Dementia*
4. *Frontotemporal Dementia (FTD)*
5. Alzheimer's Related Dementias
6. *Prevent or Slow Dementia*

The Best Science in Everyday Language

The text in both series contains American, Australian, British, and other English. I write in American English, but the research comes from the best studies worldwide. Quotes from the UK, Australia, and other English-speaking countries depend on the local dialect. For integrity, I do not edit quotes.

The books include facts and science as they exist. As much as possible, we replace medical jargon with everyday language.

Having explained the series, let's discuss dementia.

I. DEMENTIA

In this section, we discuss dementia.

Dementia is not a disease but a medical condition. Hundreds of diseases and disorders lead to dementia, but percentage-wise, almost all dementia falls under 19 primary dementia categories.

This series is the first to cover all 19 primary dementia types.

In this chapter, we answer the following questions:

- What is dementia?
- What are the 19 primary dementias?
- How prevalent is dementia?
- Who is most likely to get dementia?
- What are the financial costs to individuals, the U.S., and worldwide?

Once we answer these questions and provide a dementia overview, we turn our attention to the subject matter for the rest of the book.

Let's begin by answering the question: What is dementia?

Chapter 1: WHAT IS DEMENTIA?

For centuries, when one got dementia, people described the person in terms like "gone mad," or "lost their mind," or "crazy," or another derogatory term that missed the mark.

While most dementia types attack cognitive skills and cause behavioral disorders, the person is no less a victim than a cancer patient.

Whereas cancer attacks cells and organs, dementia destroys brain neurons.

The brain is complex. One-hundred billion neurons use over 100 trillion synapses and about 100 neurotransmitters to send all the signals to other parts of the brain, organs, and parts throughout the body, allowing us to think, reason, walk, talk, breathe, and do all that makes us human.

When fed, protected, and healthy, neurons perform magic.

The different dementias attack the brain and destroy the communication network responsible for everything our body does. By attacking different parts of the brain, the dementia types cause different disorders.

Let's see how some of the most prestigious American and global medical organizations define Dementia.

Alzheimer's Association Definition

Let's begin with the Alzheimer's Association:

> *Dementia is an overall term for diseases and conditions characterized by a decline in memory, language, problem-solving, and other thinking skills that affect a person's ability to perform everyday activities. Memory loss is an example. Alzheimer's is the most common cause of dementia*[1].

Dementia is to Alzheimer's, dementia with Lewy bodies,

Parkinson's dementia, vascular and the other dementia types what Asia is to China, India, North Korea, South Korea, and the rest of Asia. Alzheimer's is the most prevalent dementia, but each type devastates, and most are death sentences.

Let's turn to the National Institute on Aging (NIH) and see how they define dementia.

National Institute on Aging (NIH)

The National Institute on Aging (NIH) funds many studies and provides researchers invaluable data. How do they define dementia?

Dementia is the loss of cognitive functioning – thinking, remembering, and reasoning – and behavioral abilities to such an extent that it interferes with a person's daily life and activities. These functions include memory, language skills, visual perception, problem-solving, self-management, and the ability to focus and pay attention. Some people with dementia cannot control their emotions, and their personalities may change. Dementia ranges in severity from the mildest stage, when it is just beginning to affect a person's functioning, to the most severe stage, when the person must depend completely on others for basic activities of living[2].

One of the most important things a person and their loved ones can do when diagnosed with dementia; enjoy what quality time remains.

Early diagnosis, medication, and lifestyle changes can slow the disease and extend quality life. From the point of diagnosis, make the most of each good day or moment.

Let's see how the international community defines dementia.

Alzheimer's Society UK

The Alzheimer's Society is perhaps the UK's most

prestigious Alzheimer's organization. They define dementia:

> *The word 'dementia' describes a set of symptoms that may include memory loss and difficulties with thinking, problem-solving or language. These changes are often small to start with, but for someone with dementia they have become severe enough to affect daily life. A person with dementia may also experience changes in their mood or behaviour*[3].

Let's see how the World Health Organization (WHO) defines dementia.

World Health Organization (WHO)

The World Health Organization (WHO) works with global medical organizations and provides researchers a wealth of information. How does WHO define dementia?

> *Dementia is a syndrome – usually of a chronic or progressive nature – in which there is deterioration in cognitive function (i.e. the ability to process thought) beyond what might be expected from normal ageing. It affects memory, thinking, orientation, comprehension, calculation, learning capacity, language, and judgement. Consciousness is not affected. The impairment in cognitive function is commonly accompanied, and occasionally preceded, by deterioration in emotional control, social behaviour, or motivation*[4].

The four organizations provide similar definitions, each emphasizing different points, but none contradicting the others.

Each organization confirms dementia is a broad neurological disorder. Hundreds of pathologies such as Alzheimer's leads to dementia, but 19 primary types cause about 99% of dementia cases. Dementia attacks the brain and causes memory decline, behavior disorders, motor decline, language deterioration, and most types are incurable.

If doctors diagnose you with dementia, you must get past the shock. Time is moving against you, so make the most of it.

As the Alzheimer's Society points out, the symptoms are minor in the beginning. Get your affairs in order, enjoy loved ones, and take part in as many activities as you desire and are able. To some extent, this is your farewell tour. Take advantage!

The disease will stop you or a loved one later, so do not stop living your life in the early stages.

Let's next examine the 19 primary dementia types.

Chapter 2: WHAT ARE THE 19 PRIMARY DEMENTIAS?

Hundreds of medical conditions lead to dementia, but 19 causes up to 99% of cases.

Each dementia type is devastating, most are fatal, and the first symptoms to death is a challenging, heartbreaking, soul-crushing experience. Dementia robs the personalities and functionality of marvelous people a little at a time until they no longer resemble the person they've always been.

19 Dementia Types

This chapter divides the 19 primary dementias into six categories. The first group includes dementias related to Lewy body or Parkinsonism dementia. The second consists of Alzheimer's-related dementia. In the third, we focus on primary progressive aphasia dementias. The fourth contains vascular dementias. The fifth category encompasses the remaining dementias and is called *other dementias*.

Lewy Body/Parkinsonism Related Dementias

1. *Dementia with Lewy Bodies*
2. *Parkinson's Disease Dementia*
3. Corticobasal Syndrome

Alzheimer's Related Dementias

4. Typical Alzheimer's Disease
5. *Posterior Cortical Atrophy*
6. *Down Syndrome with Alzheimer's*
7. *Limbic-predominant Age-related TDP-43 Encephalopathy (LATE)*
8. Early-onset Alzheimer's

Frontotemporal Lobar Degeneration Related Dementias

9. *Behavioral Variant Frontotemporal Dementia*
10. Progressive Supranuclear Palsy

Primary Progressive Aphasia Related Dementias

11. *Nonfluent Primary Progressive Aphasia (nfvPPA)*
12. Logopenic Progressive Aphasia (LPA)

Vascular Dementia

13. *Cortical Vascular Dementia*
14. *Binswanger Disease*

Other Dementias

15. *Normal Pressure Hydrocephalus*
16. *Huntington's Disease*
17. *Korsakoff Syndrome*
18. *Creutzfeldt-Jakob Disease*
19. Amyotrophic Lateral Sclerosis

Chapter 3: WHO IS MOST LIKELY TO GET DEMENTIA?

In this chapter, we explore who is most likely to get dementia. Most know people with dementia are old, but some people are born with dementia, others get it as infants, and the disease attacks people in every age group.

There are risk factors that affect everybody. Examples include a poor diet, lack of exercise, diabetes, obesity, high blood pressure, and factors under and beyond our control.

In this chapter, we focus on risk factors affecting specific groups of people who suffer higher rates.

The research pointed to age, race, and sex, where dementia seems to discriminate. Let's review the science for each.

Age

Age is the obvious risk factor. We know because of science and our observations.

So associated with the elderly, many believe dementia only strikes older people. However, dementia strikes all ages and demographics, including newborns and infants.

According to Stanford University Medical School, "The risk of Alzheimer's disease, vascular dementia, and several other dementias goes up significantly with advancing age[5]."

None of us enjoy aging. We must work harder and harder to slow aging, and no matter how well we do, none of us will make it much past 100 years. The better we take care of ourselves, the higher chance we have of living a quality life into our eighties or nineties.

Remember, aging does not destroy our cognitive abilities. Bad habits do! I stress this point because each of us can slow the aging process through healthy habits.

As people age, however, our dementia risks increase.

A Journal of Neurology, Neurosurgery, & Psychiatry study concluded[6]:

> *In the age group 65–69 years, there are more than two new cases per 1000 persons every year. This number increases almost exponentially with increasing age, until over the age of 90 years, out of 1000 persons, 70 new cases of dementia can be expected every year.*

As we stress in our book on prevention, there is actual age and real age. We determine one's actual age by the day and year born, whereas weight, blood pressure, blood sugar, cholesterol, diet, how often you work out, and several other important factors govern our real age.

Unless genes or an accident prevents us, our real age should be lower than our actual age. Those who practice bad habits, however, raise their real age ten years or more than their actual age.

When our real age is lower than our actual age, we lower our risks for dementia and other diseases. When our real age is higher than our actual age, we increase risks for dementia, heart disease, cancer, and all major diseases.

Let's next review if race plays a role in dementia.

Race

African Americans and blacks in western countries suffer more than their share of racism.

The United States has abused too many citizens since its creation, but none more than Native Americans and African Americans.

But, does dementia also discriminate against them?

According to AARP, African Americans are 64% more likely to get dementia than non-Hispanic whites[7].

Kaiser Permanente Study

Researchers in another study examined data from 274,000 Kaiser Permanente patients over 14 years. They found the highest rate of dementia for African Americans and Native Americans[8].

Dementia Risk Per 1,000 People

- 27 African Americans
- 22 Native Americans
- 20 Latinos and Pacific Islanders
- 19 White Americans
- 15 Asian-Americans

Does dementia love Asian and European-Americans and hate African and Native-Americans?

Dementia is as evil as the worst bigot, but dementia is not a bigot.

African Americans experience higher rates of diabetes. African Americans and Native Americans suffer a higher level of stress, poverty, and disenfranchisement. Both cultures also struggle with their people's history in European-America and endure a greater level of bigotry and more obstacles to succeeding in modern America.

On the flip side, Asian Americans and whites have lower obesity and diabetes rates, eat a more balanced diet, faceless bigotry, are more affluent, educated, and successful in modern America.

We need more studies to confirm the exact causes of higher dementia incidence in the African and Native American populations. Higher stress and diabetes in their communities are prime suspects.

Jennifer Manly, Columbia University, Taub Institute for Research on Alzheimer's disease, and Aging Brain spoke to Reuters about the inequities.

There are huge disparities in dementia that are confronting this nation, and this will translate into an enormous burden on families if we don't address this. We need to prioritize research that uncovers the reasons for these disparities and more research should include racially and ethnically diverse people[9].

Are African British at a greater risk for Dementia?

In the United Kingdom, black women are 25% more likely than white women, and black men 28% more likely than white men to get dementia[10].

Reluctance to Take Part in Dementia Studies

African Americans and Native Americans are also less trustful in studies. Too often in the past, a bigoted establishment treated African Americans and Native Americans like lab rats.

The awful past makes the average African American reluctant to take part in studies that might help us figure out how to lower the rates.

Native Americans are also distrustful of the United States government and the "white man's studies," as one group from the Cherokee Reservation in North Carolina told me.

I understand both ethnic groups' skepticism. As somebody with ancestors who died and survived the Trail of Tears, and who married a black woman (30+ years), nobody must convince me of the tainted American history. I have read about the past and viewed enough with my own eyes to know the sins of America's past, either haunt or still torment today.

But, the Studies are Necessary!

I call on African Americans and Native Americans to take part in dementia studies. The studies today have greater safeguards than the past and face much more scrutiny.

Dementia is a death sentence!

Worse than the average killer, never content to kill and

move on, dementia is a sadist. Dementia destroys the mind and body, little by little, robbing one's personality, dignity, mind, body, and everything that makes a person unique.

If African Americans and Native Americans refuse to participate in dementia studies, fatal neurological disorders will continue to strike them worse than other ethnic groups.

Please consider two facts.

If you do not have dementia, researchers do not subject you to drug trials but accumulate data to determine which habits increase and decrease one's risks.

If doctors diagnose you with dementia, trials represent your last best chance to win what is otherwise a losing battle.

What Role does Poverty Play?

Although not listed as a dementia risk factor, poverty increases one's risk for almost every significant disease. Those at the bottom must worry where the next meal is coming, if somebody might mug (or kill) them when leaving the house, and a laundry list of stress the average citizen seems oblivious.

Beller Health calls for more research to determine if Native American, African American, and African British citizens have higher dementia rates as a general population, or if poverty drives these numbers. We need to know whether the number also applies to middle-and upper-class African Americans and Native Americans who eat healthily, exercise, do not abuse alcohol, avoid tobacco, and do not abuse prescription or illicit drugs.

Native American, African American, and African British citizens suffer a higher percentage of poverty than other demographics in the US and UK.

Rather than race, such factors as poverty, bigotry, and lack of opportunities might drive these numbers.

I reached out to several organizations, including the VA, to conduct a large-scale study to determine what role poverty plays in dementia. Most organizations greeted my request with enthusiasm, and I hope one or more soon back the study.

All we know for certain is poverty in the industrial world causes a much greater level of stress and other hardships than the rest of the population. WHO reported that about 60% of dementia cases occur in the poorest half of countries[11].

Age and ethnicity are dementia risk factors. What about sex?

Sex

Dementia strikes older people, African Americans, Native Americans, and African British in greater numbers than the rest of the population. Does one's gender increase or decrease one's odds?

How Many Women have Dementia?

According to the Alzheimer's Association, women represent two-thirds of people living with Alzheimer's, and 13 million women suffer dementia or are caring for somebody who does[12].

Of the 820,000 people living with dementia in the UK, females account for 61 percent[13].

Of the 50 million people living with dementia worldwide[14], women represent 65 percent[15].

Key points:

- Women represent two-thirds of Alzheimer's cases.
- Females account for 65% of dementia cases.

Is dementia just another woman-hating predator?

Does Alzheimer's & Most Dementia Strike Women in Greater Numbers?

While the two key numbers suggest dementia is a rampaging woman-abusing murderer, the answer is not so simple.

While women represent two-thirds of Alzheimer's cases and 65% of dementia cases, there are 19 primary dementia types.

Some dementias attack men in greater numbers and much harder than females. The dementias we know attack men in greater ratios include[16]:

- Parkinson's dementia (Lewy body dementia)
- Dementia with Lewy bodies (Lewy body dementia)
- Post-Stroke dementia (Vascular dementia)
- Multi-infarct dementia (Vascular dementia)
- Binswanger Disease(Vascular dementia)
- Normal pressure hydrocephalus
- Behavioral variant frontotemporal dementia
- Primary Progressive Aphasia (Frontotemporal dementia)
- Chronic traumatic encephalopathy
- HIV-related cognitive impairment
- Amyotrophic lateral sclerosis

From the data about the 19 primary dementias, at least eleven attack men in greater numbers. Data is not available for Creutzfeldt-Jakob disease, Wernicke-Korsakoff Syndrome, LATE, and Down syndrome with Alzheimer's disease. The remaining dementias strike both genders in similar numbers. When the authorities release more information, we will update this section.

If a minimum of 11 of 19 dementia types strike men in greater numbers than women, how can 68% of people living with dementia be women?

Alzheimer's accounts for 60-80% of dementia, and two-thirds of people with Alzheimer's are women.

When we say dementia attacks, women, 65% to 35% men, we distort the picture. I call on the medical community to provide greater clarity. Instead, we should warn women to represent two-thirds of total Alzheimer's cases, but stress a minimum of 11 of 19 dementia types strikes men in greater numbers.

Treating dementia and Alzheimer's as interchangeable terms is misleading. There are 19 primary dementias and 11 or more attack men in greater numbers. If we exclude Alzheimer's and focus on the other 18 primary dementia types, they attack men by far greater percentages.

With that stipulation, let's explore why Alzheimer's and some dementias attack women more than men.

Why Does Alzheimer's & Dementia Strike Women in Greater Numbers Than Men?

In part, unique burdens & responsibilities explain the disparity.

Women still fight today for equality. Like Native Americans, African Americans, and African British, the average woman carries burdens; the average man is clueless.

To be a woman, one fights for equality from birth in a "man's world," as the song and tradition attest. Among things unique to women:

- Menstrual cycles (ranging from mild to horrendous)
- Childbirth
- Menopause

Being a guy is also difficult, but there's no denying women are born with unique responsibilities and burdens.

As an aunt once retorted, if they live long enough, every woman suffers menstrual cycles until menopause "tortures it out."

Women Live Longer

Women outlive men in the United States and worldwide.

Worldwide, the average man lives to age 69.8, while the average woman lives 74.2 years[17]. These are the average numbers, so they fluctuate from region to region and country to country.

Let's see how these numbers compare to the United States.

Primary Progressive Aphasia Related Dementias

American Comparisons

The CDC reports the average American male lives 76 years, compared to the average American woman who lives 81 years[18].

Why Do Women Live Longer Than Men?

Although women live longer, this might result because more men abuse alcohol, tobacco, and drugs, get less sleep, work in more hazardous jobs, suffer greater casualties in war, and take unnecessary risks.

The lead author of a study published in the *British Medical Journal*, Australian neuropsychiatrist Richard Cibulskis, confirmed some of my suspicions.

> *Men are much more likely to die from preventable and treatable non-communicable diseases, such as {ischemic} heart disease and lung cancer, and road traffic accidents*[19].

Global population expert, Dr. Perminder Sachdev, confirmed my other suspicions in an interview with *Time*.

"Men are more likely to smoke, drink excessively and be overweight," Sachdev said. "They are also less likely to seek medical help early, and, if diagnosed with a disease, they are more likely to be non-adherent to treatment." Sachdev also pointed out, "men are more likely to take life-threatening risks and to die in car accidents, brawls or gunfights[20]."

Although nature perhaps installed a natural order to preserve the female population, men's reckless nature might account for the five years difference in life expectancy between the genders.

It will interest to see if the numbers change as more women become more like men. Women are assuming greater roles in war, law enforcement, and other areas where even men with healthy habits have fallen. As the societal lines between men and women blur, the difference in life expectancy should fall.

In all honorable fields of life, women should go for it. Never has there been a better time to prove the equality of the sexes.

As far as men's bad habits, my hope is women continue to show better judgment and exercise greater restraint. Women will never prove their equality by emulating men's worse habits or trying to outdo us in the stupid department.

The best men and women rise on similar foundations. However, the worst men and women also share a foundation. My hope for humans getting our act together soon hinges on the average woman being better than the average man.

Love yourselves for your unique feminine qualities. Be equal, but please do not confuse out-drinking, out-smoking, out-drugging, acting more reckless, and stupid than men with being equal. We need fewer men like that, not more women!

Chapter 4: DEMENTIA COSTS & PREVALENCE

In this chapter, we review dementia prevalence and costs to governments, the world, caregivers, and patients.

How Many People Worldwide Suffer Dementia?

According to the World Health Organization (WHO), over 50 million people suffer dementia worldwide, with 10 million new cases each year[21].

How Many Americans Have Dementia?

In the United States, 5.8 million Americans live with dementia[22], with Alzheimer's representing 70% of cases.

Let's check the UK dementia numbers.

How Many People in The UK Have Dementia?

According to the Alzheimer's Society, 850,000 people in the UK live with dementia[23].

Alzheimer's Society reports that about 70% of those living in UK care homes suffer dementia.

The numbers show Americans, British, and global citizens suffering high rates of dementia. Let's see which countries' dementia strikes the hardest.

Which Countries Have the Highest Dementia Rate?

Per World Atlas, the following ten countries suffer the highest dementia rate of deaths per 100,000 people[24]:

1. Finland
2. USA
3. Canada
4. Iceland
5. Sweden
6. Switzerland
7. Norway
8. Denmark
9. The Netherlands
10. Belgium

As we review the list, per population, dementia strikes Americans in greater numbers than any country but Finland.

Why?

There are several explanations:

- Over two-thirds of Americans are obese or overweight.
- The other countries on the list also suffer higher obesity levels than most countries not on the list.
- Because of weight issues, the countries in question suffer high rates of diabetes and high blood pressure, both dementia risk factors.
- Americans consume more prescription drugs than people worldwide. While there is no data to confirm, I suspect the other countries on the list also have greater access and use more prescription drugs than poorer countries.

- They load the western diet with salt, sugar, and white processed flours.
- The average person in western countries lives longer than those in poorer nations.
- We will add other factors once data becomes available.
- People live longer in these countries than most not on the list (the older one lives, the greater the dementia risk)

Another explanation is more misdiagnosis and no-diagnosis in poorer countries around the world. Obesity and other risk factors are also less of a problem in developing countries.

I recommend global researchers compare the ten countries on this list. By viewing the similarities between the ten, we might better pinpoint the cause for Alzheimer's and the other dementias.

If we can figure out what the citizens from the ten nations are doing wrong, we can find the cause and means of preventing dementia. While I pointed to some of the most obvious risk factors, the most important common risk factor from the ten nations might be something unexpected.

Let's now examine dementia costs.

Dementia Costs

In this chapter, we analyze dementia costs. We examine the United States and global costs, then provide estimated costs per family.

What Does Dementia Cost the United States?

More than the entire economies of Finland and 166 other countries, dementia costs the United States $277 billion per year.

What Does Dementia Cost Worldwide?

Getting credible global numbers proves difficult, if not

impossible, in any medical research. Often, the best source is the World Health Organization (WHO). They collect data from around the world and are an essential source for medical researchers.

Getting accurate dementia numbers in richer countries is difficult. In the United States and the UK, black people hesitate to take part in dementia studies or to seek medical attention for symptoms.

In richer countries, there are still too many misdiagnoses.

Thus, if we cannot get ironclad numbers in the United States, the United Kingdom, and the industrial nations, the task proves even more difficult for developing countries.

If the United States and the United Kingdom have difficulty convincing black citizens to seek medical attention for dementia symptoms, the third world faces even greater obstacles.

In the third world, most areas do well to offer their citizens basic medical care. With no urine or blood test, many regions lack resources for CAT scans, MRIs, and other expensive imaging equipment to make a diagnosis.

Without urine or blood tests, diagnosing dementia costs more than low-income people with inadequate or no insurance can afford in the richest countries.

In the United States and industrial nations, doctors often misdiagnose the other 19 primary dementias for Alzheimer's or each other.

Expecting doctors in many third world nations to diagnose dementia with inferior or no equipment is to expect miracles. If it overwhelms medical professionals in the wealthier nations, we often expect third world doctors to perform miracles. What amazes is they often do!

However, no matter how well the average third world doctor treats typical medical conditions, even if trained, impoverished circumstances deny them the necessary equipment to diagnose dementia early, if at all. My comments are not criticism.

The average doctor's job is not to diagnose or treat dementia, but they must recognize symptoms and refer the patient to neurologists. Primary care physicians are the first line of defense.

North, south, east, west, dementia overwhelms the medical community.

Having discussed the limitations, let's examine the data. While the numbers are ballpark figures, landing in the park is the keystone to estimation. In most cases, the real numbers are much higher.

According to the *World Alzheimer's Report,* global dementia costs a minimum of $1 trillion per year, and experts predict it will reach $2 trillion by 2030 if we find no cure[25].

Authorities should release new numbers over the next year, and we will update this section.

The *Alzheimer's Report* global cost estimations do not include informal care costs; another reason we consider the estimates conservative.

The Alzheimer's Report concluded:

> *Direct medical care costs account for roughly 20% of global dementia costs, while direct social sector costs and informal care costs each account for roughly 40%. The relative contribution of informal care is greatest in the African regions and lowest in North America, Western Europe and some South American regions, while the reverse is true for social sector costs.*

Whatever the real up-to-date costs, we must take action to reduce the burden on individuals and nations. If we do not invest in independent research to develop an effective urine or blood test, cure, and vaccine for each dementia type, the costs will smother economies throughout the world. The costs will cripple developing countries and destabilize the wealthiest.

We have no choice but to invest more in dementia research. No matter which country you live, your economy, security, and the health of your nation rides on us finding a cure or vaccine.

As a scientist, I find it disturbing climate change and independent dementia research are not major priorities. Most governments, businesses, and individuals who can afford to fund dementia remain MIA in the war against dementia.

Before we conclude this section, let's examine the dementia statistics side-by-side in the table below.

DEMENTIA STATISTICS

This table focuses on the number of people with dementia and the number of deaths per 100,000 among the nations chosen for comparison.

NATION	# OF PEOPLE WITH DEMENTIA	DEMENTIA DEATHS PER 100,000 PEOPLE	TOTAL COSTS (US DOLLARS)
Australia	447,115	29.61	$15 billion
Brazil	1 million +	10.71	$16.45 billion
Canadian	747,000	37.30	$10.4 billion
China	16.93 million	19.87	$69 billion
France	1.2 million	30.84	$37.91 billion
Germany	1.5 million	16.99	$57.57 billion
India	4 million	14.57	$28.38 billion
Italy	1.4 million	19.81	$29.96 billion
Japan	4.6 million	7.22	$14.8 billion
Mexico	800,000	3.62	Not available
Spain	800.000+	29.23	$19.98 million
Netherlands	280,000	39.37	$4.44 million
United States	5.8 million	44.41	$290 billion
United Kingdom	850,000	49.18	$26.3 billion

Sources: World Health Rankings[26], Alzheimer's Europe[27], NATSIM[28], Alzheimer's Society[29], Brain Test[30]

Other sources cited in the chapter.

The table comes from my book *2020 Dementia Overview*, which covers cost and prevalence among comparative nations in greater detail.

Let's next discuss the dementia costs for caregivers.

What Does Dementia Cost Volunteer Caregivers?

Although 41% make less than $50,000, American voluntary caregivers devote a minimum of 18.4 billion hours per year to dementia patients.

Worth $232 billion per year, we underrate the voluntary caregiving heroes in our fight against dementia. This total does not include lost wages for the voluntary caregiver.

According to the Northwestern Mutual C.A.R.E. Study, 67% of voluntary caregivers must cut their living to help pay for the patient's medical care, and 57% end up experiencing financial problems[31].

Adding to the costs of voluntary caregivers, they often end up sick themselves. Caring for loved ones with dementia bankrupts many.

In the early stages, the loved one can still perform most of their daily tasks but will require 24/7 care once the symptoms advance.

Imagine putting your life on hold for years to care, bathe, feed, protect, and take such a heavy load on your shoulders.

Millions of dementia families face the dilemma where the husband and wife both must work in most families to get by. You work as a couple to build stability in your own family, and then, boom, doctors diagnose one of you with dementia.

What Does Dementia Cost Dementia Patients?

When we say patient, past a certain stage in the disease, we refer to family or loved ones. A person who cannot perform daily tasks cannot manage finances, even if they have any left.

Too often, the costs drive entire families into bankruptcy because of dementia costs for a member.

Authorities estimate the average cost per dementia patient is $341,840, with families expected to cover 70 percent.

The costs devastate the average family in the industrial nations.

How are they supposed to afford it in developing countries where the average citizen makes less than one-thousand American dollars per year?

Primary Progressive Aphasia Related Dementias

Dementia Recap

Although your dementia research has just begun, you now have a decent overview of Dementia.

In Chapter One, we explored dementia. We turned to several top dementia or medical organizations and compared their definitions.

Chapter two explained Alzheimer's is to dementia what China is to Asia. We listed the 19 dementias. They include:

1. Dementia with Lewy Bodies
2. Parkinson's Disease Dementia
3. Corticobasal Syndrome
4. Typical Alzheimer's Disease
5. Posterior Cortical Atrophy
6. Down Syndrome with Alzheimer's
7. Limbic-predominant Age-related TDP-43 Encephalopathy (LATE)
8. Early-onset Alzheimer's
9. Behavioral Variant Frontotemporal Dementia
10. Progressive Supranuclear Palsy
11. Nonfluent Primary Progressive Aphasia
12. Logopenic Progressive Aphasia
13. Cortical Vascular Dementia
14. Binswanger Disease
15. Normal Pressure Hydrocephalus
16. Huntington's Disease
17. Korsakoff Syndrome
18. Creutzfeldt-Jakob Disease
19. Amyotrophic Lateral Sclerosis

Although most the dementia types share similar symptoms, enough to cause misdiagnosis, each has its unique pathology and symptoms.

In chapter three, we explored dementia prevalence in the United States, the UK, and worldwide.

Chapter four examined who is most likely to get dementia. We found Native Americans (those who greeted the first Europeans), and black citizens in the United States and the UK are more likely to get dementia than their white or Asian counterparts.

We also explored the women to men ratio. Women represent two-thirds of Alzheimer's and over sixty percent of dementia cases. We pointed out the Alzheimer's figure skews the dementia numbers because men are more likely to get a minimum of 11 of the 19 primary dementia types.

Chapter four explored the US, UK, global, patient, family, and voluntary caregivers' dementia costs. The staggering numbers are almost as frightening as the medical disorder itself.

We borrowed the following table from *2020 Dementia Overview*.

Dementia Costs & Prevalence

NATION	# OF PEOPLE WITH DEMENTIA	DEMENTIA DEATHS PER 100,000 PEOPLE	TOTAL COSTS (US DOLLARS)
Australia	447,115	29.61	$15 billion
Brazil	1 million +	10.71	$16.45 billion
Canadian	747,000	37.30	$10.4 billion
China	16.93 million	19.87	$69 billion
France	1.2 million	30.84	$37.91 billion
Germany	1.5 million	16.99	$57.57 billion
India	4 million	14.57	$28.38 billion
Italy	1.4 million	19.81	$29.96 billion
Japan	4.6 million	7.22	$14.8 billion
Mexico	800,000	3.62	Not available
Spain	800.000+	29.23	$19.98 million
Netherlands	280,000	39.37	$4.44 million
United States	5.8 million	44.41	$290 billion
United Kingdom	850,000	49.18	$26.3 billion

Sources: World Health Rankings[32], Alzheimer's Europe[33], NATSIM[34], Alzheimer's Society[35], Brain Test[36]

The table comes from 2020 Dementia Overview, which covers cost and prevalence among comparative nations in greater detail.

After reviewing the conservative numbers, and factoring in an aging population, we concluded we must find a cure before it bankrupts millions of families and overwhelms nations.

Having explained the series and introduced dementia, let's discuss the 19 primary dementia types.

II. 19 PRIMARY DEMENTIA TYPES

Why is it important to learn about the most prevalent dementias?

There are several reasons. One, the dementias share similar symptoms and—with no accurate testing—doctors often misdiagnose for one of a hundred or more other possibilities. Two, if a person gets one dementia, more often than not, they develop an overlapping second dementia type, known as mixed dementia. In some cases, three dementia types might develop in later stages.

The pathology, related-proteins, atrophy location, and the resulting symptoms determine dementia classifications.

The more we learn about dementia, dementia types, and subtypes grow.

We once thought of Alzheimer's disease as one sweeping neurological disorder, but now know there is typical Alzheimer's, behavior variant Alzheimer's, posterior cortical atrophy, Early-onset Alzheimer's, and the newest dementia category, LATE, previously misdiagnosed for typical Alzheimer's. If that is not complicated enough, there are 20-40 typical Alzheimer's types.

Depending on the pathology, the three primary progressive aphasia subtypes are either Alzheimer's or frontotemporal-related.

We know there is not one vascular dementia, but three: post-stroke dementia, multi-infarct dementia, and Binswanger disease.

There are two Lewy body dementias; Parkinson's disease dementia and dementia with Lewy bodies. There are also other Parkinson-related neurological disorders.

The series covers the 19 most prevalent dementia types. As noted, several are subtypes, but this work extends each equal status and inquiry

Besides breaking down the twenty most prevalent dementia types, we also discuss subtypes for each.

To reduce repetition, we divide the 19 dementias into the following sections.

Lewy Body/Parkinsonism Related Dementias

1. *Dementia with Lewy Bodies*
2. *Parkinson's Disease Dementia*
3. Corticobasal Syndrome

Alzheimer's Related Dementias

4. Typical Alzheimer's Disease
5. *Posterior Cortical Atrophy*
6. *Down Syndrome with Alzheimer's*
7. *Limbic-predominant Age-related TDP-43 Encephalopathy (LATE)*
8. Early-onset Alzheimer's

Frontotemporal Lobar Degeneration Related Dementias

9. *Behavioral Variant Frontotemporal Dementia*
10. Progressive Supranuclear Palsy

Primary Progressive Aphasia Related Dementias

11. *Nonfluent Primary Progressive Aphasia (nfvPPA)*
12. Logopenic Progressive Aphasia (LPA)

Vascular Dementia

13. *Cortical Vascular Dementia*
14. *Binswanger Disease*

Other Dementias

15. *Normal Pressure Hydrocephalus*
16. *Huntington's Disease*
17. *Korsakoff Syndrome*
18. *Creutzfeldt-Jakob Disease*
19. Amyotrophic Lateral Sclerosis

Let's shift the focus to the book topic, primary progressive aphasia related dementias.

III. PRIMARY PROGRESSIVE APHASIA DEMENTIAS

We cover two types of primary progressive aphasia (PPA) in the book series, one Alzheimer's dominant and the other to FTD dominant, although AD and FTD play a role in both PPA varieties.

Two PPA types:

1. Nonfluent/aggrammatical variant of primary progressive aphasia (naPPA)
2. Logopenic Progressive Aphasia (LPA)

There is also a third subtype, which we touch on in this section.

Chapter 5: WHAT IS PRIMARY PROGRESSIVE APHASIA (PPA)?

Depending on the pathology, primary progressive aphasia is either Alzheimer's-related or FTD-related. FTD is most linked to two subtypes, while Alzheimer's is predominant in the third. However, both Alzheimer's and FTD play a role in all three subtypes.

Mesulam Center for Cognitive Neurology and Alzheimer's Disease defines primary progressive aphasia:

> *Adults of any age can develop primary progressive aphasia (PPA), but it is more common in people under the age of 65. Individuals with PPA may have difficulties in word-finding, word usage, word order, word comprehension or word spelling. Other thinking skills (including memory for recent events, spatial orientation, recognizing faces and the essential features of personality) are initially preserved. The symptoms of PPA can cause limitations in professional, social and recreational activities that may affect one's overall quality of life*[37].

A good description. However, the last sentence might be an understatement of the century.

Let's compare the Mesulam description with one from Northwestern Medicine.

> *Primary progressive aphasia (PPA) is a form of cognitive impairment that involves a progressive loss of language function. Language is a uniquely human faculty that allows us to communicate with each other through the use of words.*

> *Our language functions include speaking, understanding what others are saying, repeating things we have heard, naming common objects, reading and writing. Aphasia is a general term used to refer to deficits in language functions. PPA is caused by degeneration in the parts of the brain that are responsible for speech and language.*

We've viewed how notable organizations describe PPA. While speech and communication are central components to PPA, patients also suffer a severe cognitive decline as the disorder progresses. We cover symptoms more in the PPA stages section.

An interesting characteristic of primary progressive aphasia (PPA) is one's word production increases before deteriorating, meaning loved ones and associates will not suspect a problem.

Therefore, loved ones must rely on the behavior problems associated with bvFTD to notice a problem. If a loved one does not notice, frontotemporal dementia develops undiagnosed, and the symptoms go unaddressed.

Let's next view the three PPA subtypes.

There are three primary progressive aphasia (PPA) types

1. Logopenic progressive aphasia (LPA)
2. Nonfluent-agrammatic variant primary progressive aphasia (naPPA)
3. Semantic variant primary progressive aphasia (svPPA)

The three PPA types[38] cause different symptoms, which we discuss in the next section. Once we finish our general PPA discussion, we devote a chapter to each subtype.

Primary Progressive Aphasia (PPA) Causes

Pinpointing the causes for most dementias, including FTD, confounds science.

Genetics causes one-third of frontotemporal dementia. Whereas brain injuries or strokes cause most aphasia, Alzheimer's or frontotemporal degeneration causes primary progressive aphasia.

According to the National Aphasia Association[39]:

PPA is caused by neurodegenerative diseases, such as Alzheimer's Disease or Frontotemporal Lobar Degeneration. PPA results from deterioration of brain tissue important for speech and language. Although the first symptoms are problems with speech and language, other problems associated with the underlying disease, such as memory loss, often occur later. PPA commonly begins as a subtle disorder of language, progressing to a nearly total inability to speak, in its most severe stage. The type or pattern of the language deficit may differ from patient to patient. The initial language disturbance may be fluent aphasia (i.e., the person may have normal or even increased rate of word production) or non-fluent aphasia (speech becomes effortful and the person produces fewer words). A less common variety begins with impaired word-finding and progressive deterioration of naming and comprehension, with relatively preserved articulation.

Both Alzheimer's and frontotemporal dementia cause primary progressive aphasia (PPA), distinguishing it from other neurological diseases but also explains why doctors often confuse the latter for the former.

Since years ago, including frontotemporal dementia in one of my books, I have called on the government to fund frontotemporal dementia research better. We need more research in three areas: causes, accurate and inexpensive tests, and a cure.

FTD researchers trudge along because most dementia research money goes to Alzheimer's, vascular dementia, and Lewy body dementia. I am not suggesting the top three dementias receive too much funding. They do not get enough research money either, but far more than frontotemporal dementia.

Science tells us genetics causes a third of frontotemporal dementia cases, but we know too little concerning the other two-thirds.

FTLD-TDP, FTLD-tau, & Alzheimer's Disease

Science does not know the exact cause, but researchers have identified three pathologies associated to varying degrees to each PPA subtype.

FTLD stands for frontotemporal lobar degenerations. In frontotemporal dementia discussions, we focus on FTLD-TDP (TDP-43) and FTLD-tau.

The three primary progressive aphasia pathologies:

1. FTLD-TDP (TDP-43)
2. FTLD-tau
3. Alzheimer's Disease

Understanding PPA subtypes, it is important to grasp a basic understanding of the three causes.

Since the media and science cover Alzheimer's more than the other dementias combined, I presume everybody has basic knowledge. Therefore, let's focus on FTLD-TDP and FTLD-tau.

What is FTLD-TDP (TDP-43)?

When discussing Alzheimer's, LATE, or one of the other dementias, the topic turns to protein buildup, plaques, tangles, and similar descriptions.

Like the other proteins, TDP-43 serves a vital function. Something, however, scientists do not understand, causes the protein to buildup in clumps, killing brain cells and tissue.

What is TDP-43's normal function?

In the cell nucleus, TDP-43 binds to DNA, regulates transcription, starting the first step in protein production.

The Genetics Home Reference[40] describes TDP-43.

> *This protein can also bind to RNA, a chemical cousin of DNA, to ensure the RNA's stability. The TDP-43 protein is involved in processing molecules called messenger RNA (mRNA),*

which serve as the genetic blueprints for making proteins. By cutting and rearranging mRNA molecules in different ways, the TDP-43 protein controls the production of different versions of certain proteins. This process is known as alternative splicing. The TDP-43 protein can influence various functions of a cell by regulating protein production.

The TARDBP gene is particularly active (expressed) during early development before birth when new tissues are forming. Many of the proteins whose production is influenced by the TDP-43 protein are involved in nervous system and organ development.

Genetics accounts for 20-40% of FTLD-TDP (TDP-43)[41].

TDP-43 serves a vital role in our development and health, so why is it implicated in dementia?

What goes wrong?

When TDP-43 misfolds, it causes impaired thinking and memory loss[42].

What is FTLD-tau?

Proteins are important to brain health, but devastating when something mysterious goes wrong and turns them into the neuron and syntax killers linked to dementia.

When healthy, tau performs an important role in the microtubules responsible for cells communicating with each other. Whereas healthy tau stabilizes the microtubules, unstable tau sticks and forms deposits and damages the microtubules[43].

FTLD-tau

The medical community divides FTLD-tau into four subtypes:

1. Argyrophilic Corticobasal degeneration (CBD)
2. Globular glial tauopathy (GGT)

3. Progressive supranuclear palsy (PSP)
4. Pick's disease.

FTLD-tau represents one primary progressive aphasia pathology.

"Tau (the Greek letter) is a microtubule associated protein, encoded by the gene MAPT gene on 17q21," said Dimitri P Agamanolis, M.D., from *Neuropathology*. "Normally, tau is phosphorylated and is present mainly in axons where it binds and stabilizes microtubules. In FTLDs, abnormal deposits of hyperphosphorylated tau in the form of paired helical or straight filaments are deposited in neurons and glial cells[44]."

The question science must answer: What destabilizes the tau protein? Is the initial problem the protein, or something else?

Some neurologists such as Dale Bredesen and David Perlmutter argue the zealous focus on protein rather than the actual causes is why every dementia drug trial fails. Although they are fighting the current, such neurologists argue the protein buildups are protective responses, not the cause.

Chapter 9: NONFLUENT/AGRAMMATICAL VARIANT OF PRIMARY PROGRESSIVE APHASIA (naPPA)

Also called progressive non-fluent aphasia (PNFA) shares similarities with the other two PPAs but distinguishes itself by how it attacks.

This frustrating primary progressive aphasia subtype inhibits people from saying words they know, words on the tip of their tongue. Patients also struggle to form sentences in the correct word or grammatical order.

The speech mechanism breaks down in this grammatic disorder. In most cases, tau protein buildup in the brain's anterior superior and inferior frontal-temporal sections causes the neurodegeneration.

Nonfluent-agrammatic variant primary progressive aphasia (naPPA) Causes

Also called progressive non-fluent aphasia (PNFA), nonfluent-agrammatic variant primary aphasia (naPPA) accounts for up to 30 percent of FTD.

According to the Penn FTD Center[45], misfolded tau protein buildup in gray matter neurons causes almost 70% of non-fluent-agrammatic variant primary progressive aphasia (naPPA).

In others, genetics cause protein TDP-43 buildup responsible for non-fluent-agrammatic variant primary progressive aphasia.

According to Grossman, the pathology of naPPA takes four paths[46].

- 52% FTLD-tau
- 25% Alzheimer's disease

- 19% FTLD-TDP
- 4% Other

Whereas FTLD-tau plays a smaller role in lvPPA, it is the dominant pathology for naPPA. Alzheimer's plays a lesser, but still significant role, accounting for a quarter of all cases. The opposite of lvPPA, FTLD-TDP plays a lesser role, accounting for 19% of naPPA.

naPPA Life Expectancy

According to the UCSF, the average naPPA patient lives 8-10 years once symptoms begin[47].

Who is Most Likely to get naPPA?

Another dementia that strikes people in their prime, naPPA strikes most people before age sixty.

Chapter 10: LOGOPENIC PROGRESSIVE APHASIA (LPA)

Also called Logopenic primary progressive aphasia and Logopenic variant PPA, logopenic progressive aphasia (LPA) is a primary progressive aphasia subtype. Both Alzheimer's and FTD cause LPA, but we list it as an Alzheimer's subtype because AD causes the majority of LPA cases.

Logopenic progressive aphasia (LPA)

Unlike other primary progressive aphasias, LPA's pathology, including amyloid deposits and neurofibrillary tangles, resembles Alzheimer's.

lvPPA begins with sporadic speech deficits and trouble finding the correct word. Sentence comprehension deteriorates[48].

Somebody with lvPPA understands words and their meaning, but neuron damage makes it impossible for them to move the muscles responsible for speech. As symptoms manifest, grammar deteriorates, including wrong pronouns, verb tenses, and word order.

The more difficult speech becomes, one withdraws or shortens sentences, leaving words out altogether. Instead of saying: "Tomorrow is my son's birthday," they say: "Son birthday...Tomorrow."

Longer sentences become even more chopped.

Logopenic Progressive Aphasia (LPA) Causes

What causes logopenic progressive aphasia (LPA) remains unknown. Researchers point to amyloid and tau protein accumulations in the brain like Alzheimer's, which kills brain cells and inferior parietal lobe and posterior temporal cortex shrinkage[49].

Three primary causes of Logopenic progressive aphasia (LPA)

According to Murray Grossman, Department of Neurology, University of Pennsylvania, LPA's pathology takes three paths[50].

- 50% Alzheimer's disease
- 38% FTLD-TDP
- 12% FTLD-tau

In LPA, Alzheimer's causes half of the cases, while FTLD-TDP causes 38% and FTLD-tau only 12% of incidents.

LPA Life Expectancy

We need more research, but the average Alzheimer's life expectancy is 8-10 years from diagnosis.

Who is Most Likely to get LPA?

LPA inflicts people in their 30's or 70's, but the average age is fifty. Somebody with Alzheimer's live with a higher risk of logopenic progressive aphasia (LPA) than somebody without AD.

Chapter 11: SEMANTIC VARIANT PROGRESSIVE APHASIA (svPPA)

The third PPA strips the ability to recognize single words. People suffering semantic variant primary progressive aphasia (svPPA) often cannot identify intimate faces or familiar objects[51].

They cannot answer what a remote control is and know not how to search for one. Hand them the remote, however, and they recognize and understand.

Somebody with svPPA uses a lot of filler words. Instead of saying, "I'm going to the kitchen, they might say: "I'm going in that there place."

Semantic variant primary progressive aphasia (svPPA) Causes

Scientists struggle to understand semantic variant primary progressive aphasia (svPPA) but confirm protein TDP-43 in the temporal lobes brain regions[52] responsible for language skills[53].

Dr. Grossman names three pathologies for svPPA[54].

69%	FTLD-TDP
25%	Alzheimer's disease
6%	FTLD-tau

Unlike with lvFTD and naPPA, FTLD-TDP accounts for 69% of svPPA. FTLD-tau only accounts for 6% of cases, while Alzheimer's accounts for a quarter of svPPA.

The same three pathologies cause all three subtypes, but to varying degrees. While scientists debate what causes the protein deposits and tangles, they agree the rogue protein kills the neurons.

The medical community has investigated dementia causes for decades and only found clues, creating enormous frustration and fierce debates.

svPPA Life Expectancy

According to UCSF, once diagnosed with svPPA, a person lives an average of 12 years[55].

Who is Most Likely to get svPPA?

Like other subtypes, svPPA attacks most people in their 50's, but also strikes younger and older.

PPA Recap

Primary Progressive Aphasia (PPA) is a progressive neurological disorder that attacks one's language and communication skills and leads to cognitive decline.

We learned in the previous section that primary progressive aphasia (PPA) is one of two primary frontotemporal dementia FTD) subtypes. While behavioral variant frontotemporal dementia (bvFTD) is more prevalent, primary progressive aphasia is no less brutal or devastating.

Whereas bvFTD causes severe behavioral problems, PPA destroys language and communication skills.

It is almost impossible to detect PPA in the earliest stages, in part because one's vocabulary increases before symptoms manifest. Instead of recognizing a problem, the patient and associates believe the victim is going through a mental growth period. With current technology, the initial increase in vocabulary makes early diagnosis impossible.

We identified three PPA subtypes.

1. Logopenic progressive aphasia (LPA)
2. Nonfluent-agrammatic variant primary progressive aphasia (naPPA)
3. Sementic variant primary progressive aphasia (svPPA)

Each attacks people's language, recognition, and communication skills.

Of the three subtypes, LPA includes amyloid protein buildups and neurofibrillary pathology, and most resemble Alzheimer's. LPA causes speech deficits. A person struggles to find the correct word to express their thoughts. LPA also diminishes sentence comprehension.

naPPA attacks somewhat different than LPA or svPPA, as patients suffer communication breakdowns, including speaking the wrong word or grammatical order.

svPPA strips one's ability to recognize words. Often, the

disorder makes it impossible to recognize familiar faces and objects.

The more we study other dementia types, we realize Alzheimer's is often also present, and in PPA's case, as the pathological prompt.

The pathology differs for each subtype.

In lvPPA, Alzheimer's causes half of the cases, while FTLD-TDP causes 38% and FTLD-tau only 12% of incidents.

Whereas FTLD-tau plays a smaller role in LPA, it is the dominant pathology for naPPA. Alzheimer's plays a lesser, but still significant role, accounting for a quarter of all cases. FTLD-TDP plays a lesser role, accounting for 19% of naPPA.

FTLD-TDP accounts for 69% of svPPA, while Alzheimer's causes a quarter and FTLD-tau only 6% of cases of svPPA.

Although evidence is lacking, I believe LATE (the newest dementia category) is also a contributor because of the TDP-43 association. LATE affects a significant part of the senior population, and until July 2019, doctors misdiagnosed LATE for Alzheimer's. I have requested the VA and several health organizations conduct studies to confirm my hypothesis.

Logopenic progressive aphasia (LPA)

The other two primary progressive aphasias show an FTD pathology. In contrast, LPA's pathology includes amyloid deposits and neurofibrillary tangles, resembling Alzheimer's.

LPPA begins with sporadic speech deficits and trouble finding the correct word. Sentence comprehension deteriorates[56].

Somebody with LPA understands words and their meaning, but neuron damage makes it impossible for them to move the muscles responsible for speech. As symptoms manifest, grammar deteriorates, including wrong pronouns, verb tenses, and word order.

The more difficult speech becomes, one withdraws or shortens sentences, leaving words out altogether. Instead of saying: "Tomorrow is my son's birthday," they say: "Son birthday...Tomorrow."

Longer sentences become even more chopped.

Semantic variant primary progressive aphasia (svPPA)

The third PPA strips the ability to recognize single words. People suffering semantic variant primary progressive aphasia (svPPA) often cannot identify intimate faces or familiar objects[57].

They cannot answer what a remote control is and know not how to search for one. Hand them the remote, however, and they recognize and understand.

Somebody with svPPA uses a lot of filler words. Instead of saying, "I'm going to the kitchen, they might say: "I'm going in that there place."

IV. PRIMARY PROGRESSIVE APHASIA DEMENTIA SYMPTOMS

This section focuses on primary progressive aphasia symptoms. We break the symptoms down for each subtype.

1. Logopenic progressive aphasia (LPA)
2. Nonfluent-agrammatic variant primary progressive aphasia (naPPA)
3. Semantic variant primary progressive aphasia (svPPA)

In the 19 dementia types section, we showed Alzheimer's is the predominant pathology of LPA and frontotemporal degeneration for naPPA and svPPA. However, Alzheimer's and frontotemporal degeneration both cause all three subtypes to various degrees.

Chapter 6: PRIMARY PROGRESSIVE APHASIA (PPA) SYMPTOMS

General PPA symptoms include:
- Can no longer grasp day-to-day things
- Declined object recognition
- Impaired person recognition
- Loses the ability to follow conversations
- No longer understands word meanings
- Reading decline
- Severe grammar decline
- Writing decline

As they differ in pathologies, the three PPA symptoms differ from each other.

Let's examine the symptoms for the three primary progressive aphasia (PPA) types.

Chapter 7: LOGOPENIC PROGRESSIVE APHASIA (LPA) SYMPTOMS

Logopenic progressive aphasia (LPA) symptoms are more related to word and phrase repetition, trouble finding the correct word, sentence, and word comprehension, and spelling, and reading.

- Grammar decline
- Impaired speech sound
- Impaired object knowledge
- Inability to comprehend or remember words
- Repeating words, phrases, and sentences
- Trouble finding the correct word

We will discuss these symptoms more in the stages section. First, let's list the symptoms for the other two subtypes.

Chapter 8: NONFLUENT-AGRAMMATIC VARIANT PRIMARY PROGRESSIVE APHASIA (naPPA) SYMPTOMS

Grammar, motor skills, and sentence comprehension are more common in nonfluent-agrammatic variant primary progressive aphasia (nfvPPA).

- Pronunciation problems
- Reduced object recognition
- Slow, broken speech
- Speech requires greater effort
- Syntactic impairment
- Word comprehension impairment
- Unusual grammar problems

Before expanding more on the subject in stages, let's cover the last PPA subtype's symptoms.

Semantic Variant Primary Progressive Aphasia (svPPA) Symptoms

In comparison, Semantic variant primary progressive aphasia (svPPA) impairment includes word recognition, spelling reading, people, object, and single-word recognition.

svPPA symptoms:

- Can no longer grasp day-to-day things
- Declined object recognition
- Impaired person recognition
- Loses the ability to follow conversations
- No longer understands word meanings
- Reading decline
- Severe grammar decline
- Writing decline

PPA Symptom Sources: Penn Frontotemporal Degeneration Center[58], *PubMed*[59], *PubMed*[60], *PubMed*[61]

Chapter 39: PRIMARY PROGRESSIVE APHASIA-RELATED DEMENTIA SYMPTOMS RECAP

Dementias share several similarities, complicating diagnosis.

- Cognitive
- Psychological (including emotional and behavior)
- Motor
- Language
- Visual/Perception

The tables help doctors and patients narrow down the possibilities when diagnosing the 19 primary dementias accounting for 99% of dementia.

All three primary progressive aphasia (PPA) subtypes produce mostly language or communication problems, with a couple of cognitive issues. Let's see how the three subtypes compare.

Primary Progressive Aphasia Symptoms

LANGUAGE SKILLS & COGNITIVE SYMPTOMS	LPA	nfvPPA	svPPA
Cannot grasp day-to-day things	X		X
Forgets familiar words	X		
Comprehension problems	X		
Grammar decline	X	X	
Impaired object knowledge	X	X	
Impaired person recognition			X
Impaired speech sound	X		
Pronunciation problems		X	
Repeats words and phrases	X		
Slow, broken speech		X	
Speech requires great effort		X	
Speech sound decline	X		
Struggles to find the correct word	X		
Syntactic impairment		X	
Word comprehension problems	X	X	
Word meaning decline			X
Writing decline			X

LPA = Logopenic progressive aphasia

nfvPPA = nonfluent-agrammatic variant primary progressive aphasia

svPPA = Semantic variant primary progressive aphasia

V. PRIMARY PROGRESSIVE APHASIA RELATED STAGES

Let's now view how the symptoms progress in stages.

Chapter 9: EARLY STAGE PRIMARY PROGRESSIVE APHASIA (PPA)

Life expectancy once PPA symptoms begin is 3-12 years[62]. In this chapter, we examine how symptoms advance through stages. Scholars and researchers break the stages into three: early-stage, middle-stage, and end-stage.

Whereas cognitive deterioration manifests in bvFTD, primary progressive aphasia attacks language skills. For most, memory and intellect remain intact in early-stage PPA.

Early Stage PPA

PPA patients suffer aphasia (language ability) and speech deterioration during the first two years, but mental functions and daily activities otherwise remain unchanged. In early-stage, aphasia is the most prevalent deterioration.

Other possible Early Stage PPA Symptoms

- Arithmetic decline
- Can no longer grasp simple words
- Difficulty following or grasping conversations
- Mispronunciation
- Reading degeneration
- Spelling deterioration
- Substituting a wrong word
- Write or speak sentences in the wrong word order

For most PPA patients, the listed symptoms evolve less prominent than aphasia deterioration.

Early-stage Logopenic progressive aphasia (LPA)

If the other two primary progressive aphasia types are atypical frontotemporal dementia, then logopenic progressive aphasia (LPA) is an atypical Alzheimer's disease (AD)[63].

Whereas the frontotemporal PPAs exhibit behavior problems similar to bvFTD, but logopenic progressive aphasia (LPA) do not.

LPA shows protein buildup in the left temporal lobe consistent with AD[64]. Cerebrospinal fluid (CSF) tests in logopenic progressive aphasia (LPA) confirm Alzheimer's patterns[65].

In early-stage LPA, a person's speech remains normal for extended periods but pauses to search the correct word[66]. Pauses grow more frequent and disturbing as the disorder progresses[67].

Somebody with early-stage LPA often hesitates and speaks slower than usual. When asked to name something, or when searching for longer words or phrases, a person with early-stage LPA. In the early stage, LPA patients also struggle to articulate digits.

Unlike typical Alzheimer's, LPA patients usually do not experience cognitive and memory issues in the first stage.

Early Stage Non-fluent-agrammatic variant primary progressive aphasia (naPPA)

A young-onset neurodegenerative disorder, microtubule protein tau buildup causes most non-influent agrammatic variant primary progressive aphasia (naPPA), damaging the left anterior superior temporal and inferior frontal regions and disrupting the neuron network[68].

The damage causes grammatical and speech interruption problems. Early-stage naPPA attacks one's ability to speak. Symptoms include:

- Stutter or hesitant speech
- Grammatic deterioration
- Form words in the wrong order

NORD describes naPPA[69]:

People with the non-fluent variant will have problems speaking with proper grammar (agrammatism). They may misuse words or leave out words such as words that connect nouns and words (e.g., to, from, the). They have difficulty finding the right word when speaking. Their speech may be stilted, which is described as slow, labored, and hesitating. They often speak less than they used to. Affected individuals also have difficulty understanding complex sentences. Sometimes individuals with this variant can have difficulty writing certain words.

Most naPPA patients maintain memory and cognitive skills in stage one. Depending on one's job and circumstances, one may continue working through stage one. The naPPA-related speech problems disrupt, disorient, and foreshadow more severe symptoms.

Early Stage Semantic variant primary progressive aphasia (svPPA)

Also considered frontotemporal degeneration, semantic variant primary progressive aphasia (svPPA) attacks the anterior and ventral temporal lobes, causing people to use the dorsal, occipitoparietal brain areas as a crutch[70].

Most svPPA patients exhibit gray matter degradation in the left anterior temporal lobe[71]. The atrophy causes conceptual and lexical loss[72].

Early-stage svPPA causes a steady decline in word recognition. Symptoms might include:

- Difficulty identifying familiar objects
- Incorrect word replacement
- Reading decline
- Spelling decline
- Talks in vague circles
- Trouble speaking
- Trouble comprehending language

Bilateral ventral temporal lobe degeneration causes concrete concept knowledge loss[73], but the inferior temporal regions remain intact[74].

Chapter 10: MIDDLE STAGE PRIMARY PROGRESSIVE APHASIA (PPA)

PPA Middle Stage

Early-stage PPA symptoms grow severe.

For many, non-aphasia symptoms (comportment and executive functions) manifest in the middle stage.

Other possible Middle Stage PPA Symptoms

- Apathy
- Facial recognition deterioration
- Foresight decline
- Improper interaction
- Object recognition decline
- Poor judgment
- Short term memory loss

Middle-stage Logopenic Progressive Aphasia (LPA)

Early-stage symptoms grow more severe. Word recognition declines and communicating becomes near-impossible.

Memory loss and other cognitive decline associated with dementia manifest in many patients.

Middle-stage Non-fluent-agrammatic variant primary progressive aphasia (naPPA)

Progressive non-fluent aphasia attacks one's ability to speak and produce language. A person can comprehend what somebody says, knows what they want to say, but naPPA strips their ability to respond.

The diagnosis of stage three takes three to four years. Middle stage naPPA limits speaking to one-word, single-words, grunts, and other inaudible noises.

In middle stage naPPA, a person keeps limited reading and writing skills, but their verbal communication declines.

Middle Stage Semantic variant primary progressive aphasia (svPPA)

Two to three years into the disease, a patient reaches middle stage svPPA. By this point, it is almost impossible to recognize names, faces, or comprehend language.

By now, svPPA patients struggle to name high visual content compared to low visual content[75].

Unlike progressive non-fluent aphasia, people with the semantic dementia version of PPA cannot read or write, but can still process shapes and colors, and comprehend numbers.

Semantic dementia attacks the brain's left side, robbing the ability to remember names for objects. Unable to remember the actual name, they create words or use filler words.

When svPPA spreads to the right side of the brain, like with bvFTD, it robs the ability to empathize, and people say or do things hurtful to others.

Chapter 11: LATE STAGE PRIMARY PROGRESSIVE APHASIA (PPA)

PPA Late Stage

Once diagnosed, the average time for PPA to reach late-stage or the "end-stage" is 4.5-5.5 years. Also called "end-stage," late-stage aphasia symptoms grow severe enough to limit speaking to single words or grunts. Many become mute by or during the late stage.

Besides limited or nonexistent communication skills, all three subtypes cause more traditional dementia symptoms such as memory loss and behavioral issues.

Comprehension and communication decline cause adverse emotions ranging from acute apathy to unbearable agitation.

In late-stage PPA, all subtypes require continuous care. At some point, families should summon hospice to help when the end is near, and the priority becomes to provide as much comfort as possible.

The apathy from earlier stages grows severe, and patients often act out in intense aggression.

We discuss subtypes as one in the final stages because they share similar symptoms by now. Patients develop a unique set of symptoms but include some combination of the following.

Possible Late Stage Symptoms

Behavioral Symptoms

- Aggression (acute)
- Agitation (severe)
- Speech limited to one word or grunt
- Unmotivated

Language & Speech Symptoms

- A decline in understanding written and spoken

language
  - Inarticulate

Motor Symptoms
  - Dexterity loss
  - Parkinson's symptoms including muscle stiffness and rigidity
  - Stiff, slow movement

Cognitive Symptoms
  - Executive decline makes it impossible to manage finances or make complex decisions
  - Oblivious of current or social events
  - Judgment decline worsens

Other Symptoms
  - Continence problems grow more severe
  - Malnourishment because of swallowing difficulty
  - Requires help with all daily tasks including eating, bathing, and dressing

The final stage lasts 1.5-2.5 years for most PPA patients. Unable to communicate themselves, nor understand others, they now must also endure declining memory and other dementia-related cognitive issues.

Late state PPA often causes reasoning, memory, and visual perceptual problems. In the late stage, it is not only difficult to distinguish the PPA subtypes from each other but also Alzheimer's and other dementias.

Eating and swallowing become near impossible. In the late stage, the afflicted person cannot walk or take care of themselves. Body functions often breakdown by late-stage PPA.

Assisted living becomes necessary in most cases, as patients require professional help with memory and speech. The key in late-stage is to provide patient love and comfort and to help them die with dignity. Some families can manage within the home, but many others require admittance into an assisted living facility for memory or speech.

Most Prevalent PPA Cause of Death

Towards the end, PPA patients require 24/7 care. The symptoms worsen until they become fragile and susceptible to infections, viruses, and accidents.

Late-stage PPA patients suffer falls, sometimes serious enough to speed their deterioration.

According to the Genetic and Rare Diseases Information Center, the most prevalent cause of death for PPA are pneumonia and injuries[76].

Hospice care becomes necessary towards the end, as all efforts turn towards comforting the patient.

PPA Stages Sources: National Aphasia Association[77], Cognitive & Alzheimer's Disease Center of Northwestern University[78], Mayo Clinic[79], *Dementia Aide*[80], Essential of Primary Progressive Aphasia[81], *Aphasiology*[82], *Classification of Primary Progressive Aphasia and its Variants*[83], Cleveland Clinic[84], PubMed Study[85], Tactus Therapy[86], Primary Progressive Aphasia[87], Association for Frontotemporal Degeneration[88,89,90], *Essentials of Primary Progressive Aphasia*[91], Harvard Medical School[92], Northwestern University Feinberg School of Medicine[93], American Academy of Neurology[94], Cleveland Clinic[95], Gray Matter Therapy[96], Alzheimer's Research UK[97]

VI. PRIMARY PROGRESSIVE APHASIA DEMENTIA RISK FACTORS

The section focuses on primary progressive aphasia symptoms. We cover two PPA subtypes:

1. Nonfluent variant Primary Progressive
2. Logopenic progressive aphasia (PPA)

The two subtypes carry many of the same risk factors, but the difference lies in the frontotemporal and Alzheimer's links. While both are linked to both subtypes, not to equal degrees.

Chapter 12: PRIMARY PROGRESSIVE APHASIA (PPA) RISK FACTORS

Scientists point towards four PPA risk factors.
- Family
- Learning disabilities
- Neurodegeneration
- Alzheimer's disease

Frontotemporal lobar degeneration, responsible for 50% of PPA cases, result from abnormal tau protein buildup[98]. Over 40% of frontotemporal lobar degeneration evolves into primary progressive aphasia.

Nonfluent Variant Primary Progressive Aphasia Risk Factors

- Family
- Learning disabilities
- Neurodegeneration
- Frontotemporal lobar degeneration
- Alzheimer's (lesser)

Logopenic Progressive Aphasia (LPA) Risk Factors

- Family
- Learning disabilities
- Neurodegeneration
- Alzheimer's disease
- Frontotemporal lobar degeneration (lesser)

Primary Progressive Aphasia Related Dementias

Family

Mutated GRN genes passed within families account for 40-50% of primary progressive aphasia[99].

Children of those who carry the mutated GRN gene have a 50% chance of getting PPA.

Genetics's role might not be as great as the numbers imply. Some neurologists believe environmental factors skew the numbers.

According to the Genetic and Rare Diseases Information Center, "Most cases of PPA are not caused by pathogenic variants in the GRN gene, but PPA can still run in families. In these situations, the disease is likely more common in the family because of shared genetic and environmental factors[100]."

Since we are creatures of habit, we can pass bad habits as dangerous as mutated genes.

Neurodegeneration

Mutated genes come in two forms, inherited from parents, and acquired (somatic) mutations caused by environmental factors[101]. With that distinction, we continue our neurodegeneration conversation.

Acquired mutations represent most PPA cases.

Three primary genes related to PPA

- FTLD-tau
- FTLD-TDP-43
- Alzheimer's disease

Alzheimer's disease accounts for 25% of the two most prevalent, naPPA and svPPA, and 50% of the less frequent lvPPA. The more we study other dementia types, the more we realize Alzheimer's is often also present, and in PPA's case, as the pathological prompt.

FTLD-TDP accounts for 69% of svPPA, while FTLD-tau leads to 52% of naPPA.

FTLD-tau

One path to PPA is an aberrant tau protein buildup, which causes frontotemporal lobar degeneration.

Tau helps regulate axonal transport and assemble and stabilize microtubules[102]. When mutated, tau protein accumulates and kills important brain cells responsible for language skills[103].

Dimitri P. Agamanolis[104], M.D., Neuropathology, teaches illustrated interactive courses for medical students and residents.

"Tau is a microtubule associated protein, encoded by the gene MAPT gene on 17q21," explained Agamanolis. "Normally, tau is phosphorylated and is present mainly in axons where it binds and stabilizes microtubules."

How about FTLD?

"In FTLDs," said Agamanolis, "abnormal deposits of hyperphosphorylated tau in the form of paired helical or straight filaments are deposited in neurons and glial cells."

Scientists estimate tau is present in 45% of FTLD[105].

FTLD-TDP-43

Also known as TARBP or TAR DNA-binding protein, FTLD-TDP-43 is a binding protein present in frontotemporal lobar degeneration[106]. Discovered in 2006, FTLD-TDP-13 is the main protein in the pathology of frontotemporal dementia FTD and primary progressive aphasia PPA[107].

The Genetics Home Reference provides an overview[108]:

> *The TARDBP gene provides instructions for making a protein called transactive response DNA binding protein 43 kDa (TDP-43). This protein is found within the cell nucleus in most tissues and is involved in many of the steps of protein production. The TDP-43 protein attaches (binds) to DNA and regulates an activity called transcription, which is the first step in the production of proteins from genes. This protein can also bind to RNA, a chemical cousin of DNA, to ensure the RNA's stability. The TDP-43 protein is involved in processing molecules called messenger RNA (mRNA), which serve as the genetic blueprints for making proteins. By cutting and rearranging mRNA molecules in different ways, the TDP-43 protein controls the production of different versions of certain proteins. This process is known as alternative splicing. The TDP-43 protein can influence various functions of a cell by regulating protein production.*

As the Genetics Home Reference stated, TDP-13 performs a positive role unless it accumulates in abnormal levels killing brain cells and tissue, which causes PPA and other neurological disorders.

Australian researchers led a study to determine FTLD-TDP-43 presence in frontotemporal dementia (FTD), including primary progressive aphasia. The study found FTLD-TDP-13 present in the hypoglossal nucleus severe enough for them to predict FTD or PPA with 99% accuracy[109].

While still requiring CAT scans, MRI's and other expensive imaging tests, if other studies confirm, the findings are a breakthrough in diagnosing primary progressive aphasia.

Whether habits or genes cause dementia, your habits matter either way. If your parent has the mutated GRN gene or not, your best chance to avoid primary progressive aphasia is eating a balanced whole food diet, exercise every day, and sleep 7-8 hours per night.

Even if your parent has the GRN gene, you still have at least a 50% chance to avoid dementia. Adopt the recommended lifestyle changes!

Alzheimer's-related PPA

The most prevalent dementia, Alzheimer's, connects directly or indirectly to multiple other brain disorders, including the three PPA subtypes.

In Alzheimer's, neurofibrillary tangles and amyloid plaques cause protein buildups in areas responsible for memory. In rare cases, the abnormal protein tangles and plaques accumulate in the brain area responsible for language skills. Up to 30% of PPA cases result from this aberrant Alzheimer's variation[110].

"PPA due to AD may be referred to as an 'atypical' consequence of AD," according to the Mesulam Center for Cognitive Neurology and Alzheimer's Disease.

PPA-related Learning disabilities

Following other studies suggesting childhood learning disabilities increased one's PPA risk, the National Institute of Health and Taub Institute for Research on Alzheimer's and the Aging Brain cosponsored a study to determine childhood learning disabilities associated with primary progressive aphasia.

The researchers compared adults who had childhood learning disabilities to those who did not. They found those who had childhood learning disabilities carried a much higher risk for primary progressive aphasia[111].

Another team of researchers from Neurology Sciences, Rush University Medical Center, tested to determine if primary progressive aphasia patients have a greater history of learning disabilities than other types of dementia and healthy people. They discovered PPA patients were much more likely to have suffered childhood learning disabilities[112].

"The patients with PPA and their first-degree family members had a significantly higher frequency of LD (learning disability) compared with the other dementia groups and the controls.," the Rush neurologists reported.

A research team from Cornell Medical College, University of Columbia School of Medicine, and Boston University School of Medicine collaborated on a case study and examined 678 "comprehensive neuropsychological assessments."

They concluded childhood learning abilities "may predispose to atypical phenotypes[113]."

Zackery Miller, MD, and colleagues from the UCSF Memory and Aging Center reviewed 279 medical records to determine if mathematical, language, or visuospatial learning deficits increase the risk of PPA.

"Nonlanguage mathematical and visuospatial LDs were associated with focal, visuospatial predominant neurodegenerative clinical syndromes," said Miller. "This finding supports the hypothesis that neurodevelopmental differences in specific brain networks are associated with phenotypic manifestation of later-life neurodegenerative disease[114]."

We must address and treat learning disabilities in children or adults to help in the short term but also reduce the risk of PPA and other neurodegenerative syndromes down the road.

VII. BONUS SECTION

Whether diagnosed with dementia or preparing for a rainy day, there are basics everybody should consider.

This section focuses on steps dementia patients (all adults) should address, including forming a care team and understanding various therapy.

While written for dementia patients, I recommend every adult fulfill these tasks before you turn thirty. Waiting is our enemy for these two duties. Be prepared!

The section includes:

1. A starter to-do list for any adult diagnosed with a fatal disease such as dementia.
2. A care team plan.

Chapter 13: Starter To-do List for Somebody and Family once Diagnosed with Dementia.

Dementia patients, loved ones, and family must address several matters early in the disease, including care, financial decisions, living quarters, Living Will, and Power of Attorney.

While you have full or most of your cognitive skills, take care of the listed priorities before diagnosis or when diagnosed. Please do not consider the items covered in this section a complete care list, but a start you tailor to your needs.

Failure to cross these items off the list while you maintain your facilities causes much regret for patients and loved ones.

Your life is your ship, and for now, you remain the captain. Plan how your ship faces the coming storm and, when you can no longer captain the ship yourself, have it already determined who takes over the helm.

Now remains your last best chance to have a substantial say in your future.

Care

Family, loved ones, and dementia patients must make difficult decisions concerning if somebody can become the primary volunteer caregiver. While dementia patients do not require 24/7 care in the early stage, it becomes necessary in the middle to late stages.

Nobody can get through dementia without others providing years of caregiving. While rare dementias kill in months, most dementia patients live for 5-20 years, with dementia growing progressively worse.

Diagnosed with dementia or in perfect health, we all must ask ourselves who would take care of us if dementia or another devastating disorder struck, requiring long-term caregiving.

Most families cannot afford professional caregiving, and the government will not help until towards the end, so family and loved ones must.

In an ideal world, we ask ourselves these tough questions and have a plan in place should something happen. This benefits not only those diagnosed with dementia but also the heroic voluntary caregivers who will see them to the end.

Financial Decisions

There are significant financial decisions to make, and earlier, the better.

Find out how much your insurance covers and the amount you must pay. A kinder world would not burden dementia patients, nor their loved ones, with overwhelming medical care costs.

In the United States and most countries in the world, the majority of dementia costs fall on families.

How Much Does Dementia Cost the Average Family?

With no urine or blood test for most dementia types, neurologists must rely on imaging and other expensive tests, often not to diagnose dementia but to rule out other neurological disorders.

Under the best scenario, related tests, doctor visits saddle the average patient with tens of thousands of dollars in deductibles by the time the neurological team diagnoses them with dementia. For some, such as dementia with Lewy bodies, it might run much higher as it can take up to eighteen months or longer before doctors make a correct diagnosis.

Our health system tells the average person: "Sorry, you have dementia. Oh, by the way, there's the bill."

Doctors, medical professionals, hospitals, drug companies, and others involved in treating dementia must make a living. Even when we factor out overcharging and profiteering, treating dementia would remain expensive.

The average American family's health insurance has deteriorated for years, the premiums growing too high, the deductibles unaffordable, and too many not worth the paper its written, much less the monthly premiums.

Authorities estimate the average cost per dementia patient is $341,840, with families expected to cover 70 percent.

Such a disease becomes a hardship for not only the patient but also their family. The demands, financial and otherwise, on voluntary caregivers often is devastating. Make difficult financial decisions early.

Financial costs vary from one dementia to another and the treatment plan.

Living Quarters

While most dementia patients maintain independence in stage one, at some point, they require help with daily tasks. Will somebody move in with her or him? Does the patient move in with somebody else? Will it become necessary for him or her to move into an assisted living community in later stages? If so, what type?

The person diagnosed should gather loved ones and decide such matters in the beginning. Like somebody on a small island with a hurricane approaching, one must be diligent. While no man or woman can withstand such a storm, they still take precautions to protect themselves and their families.

In part because of financial considerations, most families care for the loved one in the home until symptoms grow critical. Whether a dementia patient ends up in a special need living facility is not a matter of if, but at what point for those who have access.

No matter how much love, care, and attention a voluntary caregiver or loved ones provide a dementia patient, they are ill-equipped to provide for somebody in the disorder's final stretch.

Families without access do the best they can to provide comfort for the loved one but make no mistake, the patient and family benefit if a special needs facility takes over at some point.

Which type of facility depends on which dementia and symptoms. Some dementias cause more cognitive problems, while others greater affect motor skills, some visual, and a few dementias cause more language problems. In the end, many dementias are more alike than not, as the damage to the brain spreads to other areas. Still, depending on the symptoms, different care facilities might be better than others.

Ask your neurologist or local dementia organizations about local facilities trained for your particular type. Hopefully, you live at home and maintain a normal or semi-normal life for years, but have a facility selected when the end grows near.

Living Will

Not to be confused with a Last Will and Testament that distributes assets, a living will focus on medical decisions. NOLO defines a living will.

> *A living will – sometimes called a health care declaration -- is a document in which you describe the kind of health care you want to receive if you are incapacitated and cannot speak for yourself. It is often paired with a power of attorney for health care, in which you name an agent to make health care decisions on your behalf. Some states combine these two documents into one document called an 'advanced directive.'*

It is crucial to document the dementia patient's wishes while you maintain facilities to make such decisions.

Use the Living Will to direct physicians to follow your wishes on what care you receive now and, in the future, when you might not maintain your cognitive skills.

Specify end-of-life medical treatment.

NOLO recommends prioritizing life-prolonging medical care, food, and water if you become unconscious, and palliative care, which we soon address[115].

Distribute copies of your living will to loved ones, doctors, insurance providers, and all health care facilities.

Power of Attorney

The American Bar Association describes a power of attorney:

> *A power of attorney gives one or more persons the power to act on your behalf as your agent. The power may be limited to a particular activity, such as closing the sale of your home or be general in its application. The power may give temporary or permanent authority to act on your behalf. The power may take effect immediately, or only upon the occurrence of a future event, usually a determination that you are unable to act for yourself due to mental or physical disability. The latter is called a "springing" power of attorney. A power of attorney may be revoked, but most states require written notice of revocation to the person named to act for you*[116].

It is important to establish a medical power of attorney to empower a trusted loved one to make medical decisions when a patient becomes incapable. If you do not choose the right person, you can almost count on the wrong people making important decisions down the road.

If you're in early stages dementia and reading this, you likely can still think clearly, but this changes as the symptoms worsen. The only way to protect a dementia patient's wishes when they lose their cognitive decision making is by naming a power of attorney in advance.

Once you name a power of attorney, cover some dos and don'ts. After all, you are trusting another person with your life. Like with your doctors, speak your mind while you can and let people know what you expect.

As NOLO pointed out, some states merge the living will and power of attorney into an advanced directive. Whether together or separate, I recommend all adults, and particularly those diagnosed with dementia, draw up a medical living will and name a power of attorney.

The starter to-do list provides a starting point for dementia patients, families, and any adult.

Once diagnosed, both the person diagnosed and loved ones must unite and build your to-do list. Add whatever makes sense for you and your unique situation.

Let's next cover a few key members of a dementia care team.

Chapter 14: CARE TEAM

The National Institute on Aging recommends building a care team.

The team includes an art therapist, mental health counselor, occupational therapist, palliative care specialist, physical therapist, and a speech therapist[117].

Art therapist

The art therapist reduces stress by engaging the patient in music and other expressive arts.

Since dementia causes enormous anxiety and mood swings, art therapists use music and art to soothe patients and assist caregivers. Most everybody responds to music. Some pump our blood and makes us want to shake our bodies to the rhythm. Other music helps us focus and achieve maximum concentration.

Some music geared towards dementia patients relaxes and calms. Music is a godsend!

Art is not a task but a love affair. Some say within each of us is an artist starving to escape. Art therapists use music and art as a brilliant tool to treat dementia anxiety, attention decline, sleep problems, etc.

Mental health counselors

A neurological disorder, dementia attacks the brain and inhibits cognitive skills. Mental health counselors help patients and families plan for the future and cope with the shock, hurt, and pain resulting from the diagnosis.

Most individuals and families suffer chronic mental stress when doctors diagnose a member with dementia.

Find a mental health counselor trained in dementia.

Turn to their expertise and do not allow the neurological disorder to destroy the remaining quality of life for the patient, or respond as a family in a way where dementia destroys many lives by one sweeping event.

Occupational therapists

The occupational therapist helps patients bathe, dress, eat, and perform daily tasks.

We think of the routine daily tasks as second nature, and it is as long as the neurons, pathways, arteries, heart, and brain perform as normal. When suffering a stroke or neurological disorder like dementia, we quickly learn nothing is second nature anymore. Like a child, dementia patients often must relearn how to perform basic tasks.

Occupational therapists help patients remain independent and then semi-independent, as long as possible, extending the quality of life. An occupational therapist is instrumental in treating most dementias.

Palliative care specialist

The palliative care specialist minimizes symptoms from diagnosis to the end. You or a loved one need somebody who addresses symptoms as soon as they arise, so find a quality palliative care specialist.

They extend the quality of life and reduce suffering.

Physical therapists

Physical therapists help motors skills by leading patients through exercise.

Although dementia is known as a mental disorder, what affects the brain affects the body and vice versa. Find a physical therapist trained to work with your specific dementia.

If you've seen somebody suffering Parkinsonism or other neurological disorders affecting movement, you have an idea of the problems some dementias cause, even in the earliest stages.

A physical therapist helps maintain balance and strength, allowing a person to walk and move on their own. As dementia progresses, so does the physical therapist's importance.

Speech therapists

The speech therapist addresses speech and swallowing problems, issues present in early dementia symptoms for some types, and eventually becomes a problem for most dementias.

What is the value of verbalizing one's thoughts, understanding what a loved one says, and swallowing our food without choking or causing infection by sending it down the wrong pipe?

These are issues speech therapists excel. The ones I've observed are passionate about helping people retrain the mind to overcome aphasia and swallowing problems.

Find a speech (and other types of) therapist trained in treating your specific type of dementia. These different listed therapists can minimize the long nightmare following a dementia diagnosis.

Chapter 15: LETTER TO CONGRESS

DEAR U.S. CONGRESS, NATIONS OF THE WORLD, & WEALTHY HUMANS

We call on the United States and the governments of the world to spend less on war and walls and more on Alzheimer's and dementia research.

If aliens were attacking us from another planet, I presume the nations of the world would unite against a common enemy. That is what I propose now.

The enemy I refer to does not come from another planet but threatens humans no less. Alzheimer's and dementia strike an American every 68 seconds and somebody worldwide every 30 seconds.

The nations of the world can save millions of lives and billions of dollars.

We need necessary funding to:

1. Discover the exact cause (s) of Alzheimer's and other dementias.
2. Develop accurate testing for Alzheimer's and other dementias.
3. Develop a vaccine to wipe out Alzheimer's and other dementias like we did polio.

Alzheimer's and dementia grow at a rate that will destroy the economies of most countries if we do not become more proactive.

We can save trillions of dollars for future generations if we invest now in discovering the exact cause (s), a vaccine to prevent it from happening, and other steps to defeat this horrifying disease.

Alzheimer's and other dementias threaten every family in all nations.

We can do little for those with late-stage dementia, but the proposed steps might save millions of lives and trillions of dollars by diagnosing the different dementias early and treating them before they do significant damage.

Beller Health calls on politicians, corporations, and wealthy individuals to step forward to help win the war against dementia.

CONCLUSION

Thank you for reading this book. We covered a good amount of material.

Dementia is a cruel neurological disorder that robs people of their personalities, executive skills, memories, talents, language, voice, motor capabilities, and all that makes us individual humans.

Alzheimer's and Dementia

Although Alzheimer's disease (AD) is the most prevalent, we learned AD is to dementia what China is to Asia. Alzheimer's represents 60-80% of dementia, but 19 dementia types account for 99 percent.

Dementia Spares No Demographic

Dementia's reputation is known as an old folk's disease but strikes people all ages. Most dementia is not genetic, although certain types such as Huntington's disease are 100% familial.

Most Dementia is Incurable

Most dementia is incurable, but—if caught early enough—neurosurgeons can treat and sometimes reverse normal pressure hydrocephalus.

Dementia Prevalence

The first section focused on dementia as a general category. We learned 850,000 people in the UK have dementia, compared to 5.8 Americans and 50 million people worldwide.

Dementia Categories

We divided the 19 dementias into six categories:

- Lewy Body/Parkinsonism related dementias
- Alzheimer's related dementias
- Frontotemporal lobar degeneration related dementias
- Primary progressive aphasia related dementias
- Vascular dementias
- Other dementias

19 Dementia Types

Lewy Body/Parkinsonism Related Dementias

1. *Dementia with Lewy Bodies*
2. *Parkinson's Disease Dementia*
3. Corticobasal Syndrome

Alzheimer's Related Dementias

4. Typical Alzheimer's Disease
5. *Posterior Cortical Atrophy*
6. *Down Syndrome with Alzheimer's*
7. *Limbic-predominant Age-related TDP-43 Encephalopathy (LATE)*
8. Early-onset Alzheimer's

Frontotemporal Lobar Degeneration Related Dementias

9. *Behavioral Variant Frontotemporal Dementia*
10. Progressive Supranuclear Palsy

Primary Progressive Aphasia Related Dementias

11. *Nonfluent Primary Progressive Aphasia (nfvPPA)*

12. <u>Logopenic Progressive Aphasia (LPA)</u>

Vascular Dementia

13. *<u>Cortical Vascular Dementia</u>*
14. *<u>Binswanger Disease</u>*

Other Dementias

15. *<u>Normal Pressure Hydrocephalus</u>*
16. *<u>Huntington's Disease</u>*
17. *<u>Korsakoff Syndrome</u>*
18. *<u>Creutzfeldt-Jakob Disease</u>*
19. <u>Amyotrophic Lateral Sclerosis</u>

We examined primary progressive aphasia related dementias, defining and exploring causes, prevalence, symptoms, and stages.

THE END

Of

PRIMARY PROGRESSIVE APHASIA RELATED DEMENTIAS

THANK YOU FOR READING

Thank you for reading the entire book. While this is not a literary work to enjoy, I hope you gained useful knowledge of posterior cortical atrophy.

If you benefitted from this book, please take a moment to share your thoughts in a review. Reader reviews help other readers make educated decisions about this book before purchasing.

Book Review link for Dementia Types, Symptoms, Stages, & Risk Factors

or

https://www.amazon.com/dp/B07ZG142FM

Look for annual updates to my health books, as I follow new studies and add any helpful information I find. Health and fitness are top priorities, and the heart and brain are my specialties.

I hope you develop the habits suggested in this book. Good luck on your health journey. Live long and prosper, my friend.

All the best,
Jerry Beller & Beller Health

BELLER HEALTH BOOKS

Beller Health Research Institute specializes in the heart and brain, and published the following Jerry Beller book series:

- Arrhythmia Series
- Vascular Disease Series
- 2020 Dementia Overview Series
- 19 Dementia Types Series

Please continue to view the books in each series.

Primary Progressive Aphasia Related Dementias

Dementia Types, Symptoms, Stages, & Risk Factors Series

This book series is the first to cover each of the 19 primary dementia types.

20. *Dementia with Lewy Bodies*
21. *Parkinson's Disease Dementia*
22. Corticobasal Syndrome
23. Typical Alzheimer's Disease
24. *Posterior Cortical Atrophy*
25. *Down Syndrome with Alzheimer's*
26. *Limbic-predominant Age-related TDP-43 Encephalopathy (LATE)*
27. Early-onset Alzheimer's
28. *Behavioral Variant Frontotemporal Dementia*
29. Progressive Supranuclear Palsy
30. *Nonfluent Primary Progressive Aphasia*
31. Logopenic Progressive Aphasia
32. *Cortical Vascular Dementia*
33. *Binswanger Disease*
34. *Normal Pressure Hydrocephalus*
35. *Huntington's Disease*
36. *Korsakoff Syndrome*
37. *Creutzfeldt-Jakob Disease*
38. Amyotrophic Lateral Sclerosis

2020 Dementia Overview Series

Whereas in the *Dementia Types, Symptoms, Stages, and Risk Factors* series, each book covers a different dementia type, this series focuses on groups of dementias.

1. Dementia Types, Symptoms, & Stages
2. *Lewy Body/Parkinsonism Dementias*
3. *Vascular Dementia*
4. *Frontotemporal Dementia (FTD)*
5. Alzheimer's Related Dementias
6. *Prevent or Slow Dementia*

Other Beller Health Books

You can view or purchase all Beller Health Books on Amazon at the following web address:

https://amzn.to/2TpDr8e

ABOUT THE AUTHOR

Jerry Beller is the lead author and researcher at Beller Medical Research Institute. Beller distinguished himself three times in the medical world by being the first to write and publish books on particular dementia fields.

He wrote the first book covering all 15 primary dementia types, which he since expanded to cover nineteen. Beller followed this accomplishment by writing a book on each dementia type. He broke medical ground a third time when he published the first book on the new dementia category LATE.

When the world struggled to grasp the difference between Alzheimer's disease and China, Beller explained:

> *Alzheimer's is only one dementia, much like China is only one country in Asia. Just as we do not want to ignore the other countries in Asia because China is the largest, nor do we want to ignore the less prevalent dementia types.*

Despite his accomplishments, he remains humble. "Until we win the dementia war, I've no reason to celebrate," Beller said. "If we win the war during my lifetime, I will celebrate with a few hundred brothers and sisters around the world who share my passion. Until then, we have too much work left to worry about accolades and legacies."

When not researching dementia, Jerry enjoys life with his wife of thirty-plus years, Nicola, and their two children.

Visit Jerry Beller:

https://bellerhealth.com

1 'What Is Dementia?', Alzheimer's Disease and Dementia <https://alz.org/alzheimers-dementia/what-is-dementia> [accessed 18 September 2019].

2 'What Is Dementia? Symptoms, Types, and Diagnosis', National Institute on Aging <https://www.nia.nih.gov/health/what-dementia-symptoms-types-and-diagnosis> [accessed 18 September 2019].

[3] 'What Is Dementia?', *Alzheimer's Society* <https://www.alzheimers.org.uk/about-dementia/types-dementia/what-dementia> [accessed 18 September 2019].

[4] 'Dementia' <https://www.who.int/news-room/fact-sheets/detail/dementia> [accessed 18 September 2019].

[5] 'Risk Factors' <https://stanfordhealthcare.org/medical-conditions/brain-and-nerves/dementia/risk-factors.html> [accessed 20 September 2019].

[6] W. M. van der Flier and P. Scheltens, 'Epidemiology and Risk Factors of Dementia', *Journal of Neurology, Neurosurgery & Psychiatry*, 76.suppl 5 (2005), v2–7 <https://doi.org/10.1136/jnnp.2005.082867>.

[7] Kent Allen, 'Dementia Rates to Grow for African Americans, Hispanics', *AARP* <http://www.aarp.org/health/dementia/info-2018/dementia-alzheimer-cases-grow-nonwhites.html> [accessed 20 September 2019].

[8] Elizabeth Rose Mayeda and others, 'Inequalities in Dementia Incidence between Six Racial and Ethnic Groups over 14 Years', *Alzheimer's & Dementia: The Journal of the Alzheimer's Association*, 12.3 (2016), 216–24 <https://doi.org/10.1016/j.jalz.2015.12.007>.

[9] 'African Americans at Higher Dementia Risk than Other Racial Groups', *Reuters*, 10 March 2016 <https://www.reuters.com/article/us-health-dementia-race-u-s-idUSKCN0WC2X5> [accessed 20 September 2019].

[10] Steve Ford, 'Likelihood of Dementia "Higher among Black Ethnic Groups"', *Nursing Times*, 2018 <https://www.nursingtimes.net/news/research-and-innovation/likelihood-of-dementia-higher-among-black-ethnic-groups-08-08-2018/> [accessed 21 September 2019].

[11] 'Dementia' <https://www.who.int/news-room/fact-sheets/detail/dementia> [accessed 21 September 2019].

[12] 'Women and Alzheimer's', *Alzheimer's Disease and Dementia* <https://alz.org/alzheimers-dementia/what-is-alzheimers/women-and-alzheimer-s> [accessed 21 September 2019].

[13] 'Dementia Facts', *Dementia Consortium* <https://www.dementiaconsortium.org/dementia-facts/> [accessed 21 September 2019].

[14] 'Dementia' <https://www.who.int/news-room/fact-sheets/detail/dementia> [accessed 21 September 2019].

[15] 'Why Is Dementia Different for Women?', *Alzheimer's Society* <https://www.alzheimers.org.uk/blog/why-dementia-different-women> [accessed 21 September 2019].

[16] Jessica L. Podcasy and C. Neill Epperson, 'Considering Sex and Gender in Alzheimer Disease and Other Dementias', *Dialogues in Clinical Neuroscience*, 18.4 (2016), 437–46 <https://www.ncbi.nlm.nih.gov/pmc/articles/PMC5286729/> [accessed 21 September 2019].

[17] 'WHO | Life Expectancy', *WHO* <http://www.who.int/gho/mortality_burden_disease/life_tables/situation_trends_text/en/> [accessed 21 September 2019].

[18] 'Products - Data Briefs - Number 328 - November 2018', 2019 <https://www.cdc.gov/nchs/products/databriefs/db328.htm> [accessed 21 September 2019].

[19] Jacqui Thornton, 'WHO Report Shows That Women Outlive Men Worldwide', *BMJ*, 365 (2019), l1631 <https://doi.org/10.1136/bmj.l1631>.

[20] 'Why Do Women Live Longer Than Men?', *Time* <https://time.com/5538099/why-do-women-live-longer-than-men/> [accessed 21 September 2019].

[21] 'Dementia' <https://www.who.int/news-room/fact-sheets/detail/dementia> [accessed 20 September 2019].

[22] 'Alzheimer's Disease: Facts & Figures', *BrightFocus Foundation*, 2015 <https://www.brightfocus.org/alzheimers/article/alzheimers-disease-facts-figures> [accessed 4 September 2019].

[23] 'Facts for the Media', *Alzheimer's Society* <https://www.alzheimers.org.uk/about-us/news-and-media/facts-media> [accessed 20 September 2019].

[24] 'Countries With The Highest Rates Of Deaths From Dementia',

WorldAtlas <https://www.worldatlas.com/articles/countries-with-the-highest-rates-of-deaths-from-dementia.html> [accessed 20 September 2019].

[25] 'World Alzheimer Report 2018 - The State of the Art of Dementia Research: New Frontiers', *NEW FRONTIERS*, 48.

[26] 'ALZHEIMERS/DEMENTIA DEATH RATE BY COUNTRY', *World Life Expectancy* <https://www.worldlifeexpectancy.com/cause-of-death/alzheimers-dementia/by-country/> [accessed 24 September 2019].

[27] 'Alzheimer Europe - Research - European Collaboration on Dementia - Cost of Dementia - Regional/National Cost of Illness Estimates' <https://www.alzheimer-europe.org/Research/European-Collaboration-on-Dementia/Cost-of-dementia/Regional-National-cost-of-illness-estimates> [accessed 26 September 2019].

[28] 'Publications | NATSEM' <https://www.natsem.canberra.edu.au/publications/?publication=economic-cost-of-dementia-in-australia-2016-2056> [accessed 22 September 2019].

[29] 'Dementia UK Report', *Alzheimer's Society* <https://www.alzheimers.org.uk/about-us/policy-and-influencing/dementia-uk-report> [accessed 22 September 2019].

[30] 'Dementia Statistics – U.S. & Worldwide Stats', *BrainTest*, 2015 <https://braintest.com/dementia-stats-u-s-worldwide/> [accessed 23 September 2019].

[31] 'Newsroom | Northwestern Mutual - 2018 C.A.R.E. Study', *Newsroom | Northwestern Mutual* <https://news.northwesternmutual.com/2018-care-study> [accessed 22 September 2019].

[32] 'ALZHEIMERS/DEMENTIA DEATH RATE BY COUNTRY'.

[33] 'Alzheimer Europe - Research - European Collaboration on Dementia - Cost of Dementia - Regional/National Cost of Illness Estimates'.

[34] 'Publications | NATSEM'.

[35] 'Dementia UK Report'.

[36] 'Dementia Statistics – U.S. & Worldwide Stats'.

[37] 'Primary Progressive Aphasia' <https://www.brain.northwestern.edu/dementia/ppa/index.html> [accessed 25 October 2019].

[38] INSERM US14-- ALL RIGHTS RESERVED, 'Orphanet: Primary

Progressive Aphasia' <https://www.orpha.net/consor/cgi-bin/OC_Exp.php?lng=en&Expert=95432> [accessed 28 April 2019].

[39] 'Primary Progressive Aphasia', *National Aphasia Association* <https://www.aphasia.org/aphasia-resources/primary-progressive-aphasia/> [accessed 15 January 2019].

[40] Genetics Home Reference, 'TARDBP Gene', *Genetics Home Reference* <https://ghr.nlm.nih.gov/gene/TARDBP> [accessed 6 May 2019].

[41] Edward B. Lee and others, 'Expansion of the Classification of FTLD-TDP: Distinct Pathology Associated with Rapidly Progressive Frontotemporal Degeneration', *Acta Neuropathologica*, 134.1 (2017), 65–78 <https://doi.org/10.1007/s00401-017-1679-9>.

[42] Neuroscience News, 'When Is Alzheimer's Not Alzheimer's? Researchers Characterize a Different Form of Dementia', *Neuroscience News*, 2019 <https://neurosciencenews.com/dementia-tdp-43-late-12090/> [accessed 7 May 2019].

[43] V. M. Lee, M. Goedert, and J. Q. Trojanowski, 'Neurodegenerative Tauopathies', *Annual Review of Neuroscience*, 24 (2001), 1121–59 <https://doi.org/10.1146/annurev.neuro.24.1.1121>.

[44] 'Frontotemporal Dementias' <http://neuropathology-web.org/chapter9/chapter9cFTD.html> [accessed 27 October 2019].

[45] 'The Penn FTD Center | Nonfluent/Agrammatic Primary Progressive Aphasia (Progressive Non-Fluent Aphasia)' <https://ftd.med.upenn.edu/about-ftd-related-disorders/what-are-these-conditions/progressive-language/progressive-nonfluent-aphasia-pna> [accessed 27 April 2019].

[46] Murray Grossman, 'THE NON-FLUENT/AGRAMMATIC VARIANT OF PRIMARY PROGRESSIVE APHASIA', *Lancet Neurology*, 11.6 (2012), 545–55 <https://doi.org/10.1016/S1474-4422(12)70099-6>.

[47] 'Nonfluent Variant Primary Progressive Aphasia', *Memory and Aging Center* <https://memory.ucsf.edu/dementia/primary-progressive-aphasia/nonfluent-variant-primary-progressive-aphasia> [accessed 5 December 2019].

[48] Serena Amici and others, 'An Overview on Primary Progressive Aphasia and Its Variants', *Behavioural Neurology*, 17.2 (2006), 77–87.

[49] Maxime Montembeault and others, 'Clinical, Anatomical, and Pathological Features in the Three Variants of Primary Progressive Aphasia: A Review', *Frontiers in Neurology*, 9 (2018)

<https://doi.org/10.3389/fneur.2018.00692>.

[50] Grossman, 'THE NON-FLUENT/AGRAMMATIC VARIANT OF PRIMARY PROGRESSIVE APHASIA'.

[51] Bruce L. Miller, *The Clinical Syndrome of SvPPA* (Oxford University Press) <http://oxfordmedicine.com/view/10.1093/med/9780195380491.001.0001/med-9780195380491-chapter-3> [accessed 27 April 2019].

[52] Leonardo Iaccarino and others, 'The Semantic Variant of Primary Progressive Aphasia: Clinical and Neuroimaging Evidence in Single Subjects', *PLoS ONE*, 10.3 (2015) <https://doi.org/10.1371/journal.pone.0120197>.

[53] 'Patterns of Temporal Lobe Atrophy in Semantic Dementia and Alzheimer's Disease - Chan - 2001 - Annals of Neurology - Wiley Online Library' <https://onlinelibrary.wiley.com/doi/abs/10.1002/ana.92> [accessed 27 April 2019].

[54] Grossman, 'THE NON-FLUENT/AGRAMMATIC VARIANT OF PRIMARY PROGRESSIVE APHASIA'.

[55] 'Semantic Variant Primary Progressive Aphasia', *Memory and Aging Center* <https://memory.ucsf.edu/dementia/primary-progressive-aphasia/semantic-variant-primary-progressive-aphasia> [accessed 6 December 2019].

[56] Amici and others.

[57] Miller.

[58] 'The Penn FTD Center | Semantic Variant Primary Progressive Aphasia (Semantic Dementia)' <https://ftd.med.upenn.edu/about-ftd-related-disorders/what-are-these-conditions/progressive-language/semantic-variant-primary-progressive-aphasia-svppa> [accessed 29 April 2019].

[59] Murray Grossman, 'Primary Progressive Aphasia: Clinicopathological Correlations', *Nature Reviews. Neurology*, 6.2 (2010), 88–97 <https://doi.org/10.1038/nrneurol.2009.216>.

[60] Murray Grossman, 'THE NON-FLUENT/AGRAMMATIC VARIANT OF PRIMARY PROGRESSIVE APHASIA', *Lancet Neurology*, 11.6 (2012), 545–55 <https://doi.org/10.1016/S1474-4422(12)70099-6>.

[61] M.L. Gorno-Tempini and others, 'Classification of Primary Progressive Aphasia and Its Variants', *Neurology*, 76.11 (2011), 1006–

14 <https://doi.org/10.1212/WNL.0b013e31821103e6>.

[62] Ging-Yuek Robin Hsiung and Howard H. Feldman, 'GRN-Related Frontotemporal Dementia', in *GeneReviews®*, ed. by Margaret P. Adam and others (Seattle (WA): University of Washington, Seattle, 1993) <http://www.ncbi.nlm.nih.gov/books/NBK1371/> [accessed 30 April 2019].

[63] Manja Lehmann and others, 'Intrinsic Connectivity Networks in Healthy Subjects Explain Clinical Variability in Alzheimer's Disease', *Proceedings of the National Academy of Sciences of the United States of America*, 110.28 (2013), 11606–11 <https://doi.org/10.1073/pnas.1221536110>.

[64] Jennifer L. Whitwell and others, 'Working Memory and Language Network Dysfunctions in Logopenic Aphasia: A Task-Free FMRI Comparison with Alzheimer's Dementia', *Neurobiology of Aging*, 36.3 (2015), 1245–52 <https://doi.org/10.1016/j.neurobiolaging.2014.12.013>.

[65] Edmond Teng and others, 'CEREBROSPINAL FLUID BIOMARKERS IN CLINICAL SUBTYPES OF EARLY-ONSET ALZHEIMER'S DISEASE', *Dementia and Geriatric Cognitive Disorders*, 37.0 (2014), 307–14 <https://doi.org/10.1159/000355555>.

[66] M. L. Gorno-Tempini, S. M. Brambati, and others, 'The Logopenic/Phonological Variant of Primary Progressive Aphasia', *Neurology*, 71.16 (2008), 1227–34 <https://doi.org/10.1212/01.wnl.0000320506.79811.da>.

[67] Maya L. Henry and others, 'Phonological Processing in Primary Progressive Aphasia', *Journal of Cognitive Neuroscience*, 28.2 (2016), 210–22 <https://doi.org/10.1162/jocn_a_00901>.

[68] Murray Grossman, 'The Non-Fluent/Agrammatic Variant of Primary Progressive Aphasia', 11 (2012), 11.

[69] 'Frontotemporal Degeneration', *NORD (National Organization for Rare Disorders)* <https://rarediseases.org/rare-diseases/frontotemporal-degeneration/> [accessed 8 December 2019].

[70] V. Borghesani and others, *Taking the Sub-Lexical Route: Brain Dynamics of Reading in the Semantic Variant of Primary Progressive Aphasia* (Neuroscience, 21 November 2019) <https://doi.org/10.1101/847798>.

[71] Katheryn A. Q. Cousins and others, 'Longitudinal Changes in Semantic Concreteness in Semantic Variant Primary Progressive Aphasia

(SvPPA)', *ENeuro*, 5.6 (2018) <https://doi.org/10.1523/ENEURO.0197-18.2018>.

[72] John R. Hodges and Karalyn Patterson, 'Semantic Dementia: A Unique Clinicopathological Syndrome', *The Lancet. Neurology*, 6.11 (2007), 1004–14 <https://doi.org/10.1016/S1474-4422(07)70266-1>.

[73] Matthew A. Lambon Ralph and others, 'Taking Both Sides: Do Unilateral Anterior Temporal Lobe Lesions Disrupt Semantic Memory?', *Brain: A Journal of Neurology*, 133.11 (2010), 3243–55 <https://doi.org/10.1093/brain/awq264>.

[74] Katheryn A. Q. Cousins and others, 'Longitudinal Changes in Semantic Concreteness in Semantic Variant Primary Progressive Aphasia (SvPPA)', *ENeuro*, 5.6 (2018) <https://doi.org/10.1523/ENEURO.0197-18.2018>.

[75] Karalyn Patterson, Peter J. Nestor, and Timothy T. Rogers, 'Where Do You Know What You Know? The Representation of Semantic Knowledge in the Human Brain', *Nature Reviews. Neuroscience*, 8.12 (2007), 976–87 <https://doi.org/10.1038/nrn2277>.

[76] 'Primary Progressive Aphasia | Genetic and Rare Diseases Information Center (GARD) – an NCATS Program' <https://rarediseases.info.nih.gov/diseases/8541/primary-progressive-aphasia/cases/47508> [accessed 30 April 2019].

[77] 'Living with Primary Progressive Aphasia (PPA)', *National Aphasia Association*, 2015 <https://www.aphasia.org/stories/living-with-primary-progressive-aphasia-ppa-2/> [accessed 21 January 2019].

[78] 'PPAInformation2016.Pdf' <https://www.brain.northwestern.edu/pdfs/PPA/PPAInformation2016.pdf> [accessed 21 January 2019].

[79] 'Primary Progressive Aphasia - Symptoms and Causes', *Mayo Clinic* <https://www.mayoclinic.org/diseases-conditions/primary-progressive-aphasia/symptoms-causes/syc-20350499> [accessed 21 January 2019].

[80] 'Fronto-Temporal Dementia: Where Age Is Just a Number', *Dementia Aide* <https://www.dementiaaide.com/blogs/tips-for-dementia/fronto-temporal-dementia-guide> [accessed 21 January 2019].

[81] Marsel Mesulam, 'Essentials of Primary Progressive Aphasia', 17.

[82] '26-01.Pdf' <http://eprints-prod-05.library.pitt.edu/1101/1/26-

01.pdf> [accessed 21 January 2019].

[83] M. L. Gorno-Tempini, A. E. Hillis, and others, 'Classification of Primary Progressive Aphasia and Its Variants', *Neurology*, 76.11 (2011), 1006–14 <https://doi.org/10.1212/WNL.0b013e31821103e6>.

[84] 'Primary Progressive Aphasia', *Cleveland Clinic* <https://my.clevelandclinic.org/health/diseases/17387-primary-progressive-aphasia> [accessed 21 January 2019].

[85] Daisy Sapolsky, Kimiko Domoto-Reilly, and Bradford C. Dickerson, 'Use of the Progressive Aphasia Severity Scale (PASS) in Monitoring Speech and Language Status in PPA', *Aphasiology*, 28.8–9 (2014), 993–1003 <https://doi.org/10.1080/02687038.2014.931563>.

[86] Tactus Therapy Guest Blogger, 'Primary Progressive Aphasia: Therapy Tips for the Speech-Language Pathologist', *Tactus Therapy Solutions*, 2018 <https://tactustherapy.com/ppa-treatment-slp-primary-progressive-aphasia/> [accessed 1 May 2019].

[87] 'PPA Later Stages – Rare Dementia Support' <http://www.raredementiasupport.org/ppa/ppa-later-stages/> [accessed 1 May 2019].

[88] 'Logopenic Variant PPA (Primary Progressive Aphasia)', *AFTD* <https://www.theaftd.org/what-is-ftd/primary-progressive-aphasia/logopenic-variant-ppa/> [accessed 1 May 2019].

[89] 'Nonfluent/Agrammatic PPA (Primary Progressive Aphasia)', *AFTD* <https://www.theaftd.org/what-is-ftd/primary-progressive-aphasia/nonfluent-agrammatic-ppa-nfvppa/> [accessed 1 May 2019].

[90] 'Semantic Variant PPA (Primary Progressive Aphasia)', *AFTD* <https://www.theaftd.org/what-is-ftd/primary-progressive-aphasia/semantic-variant-ppa-svppa/> [accessed 1 May 2019].

[91] Marsel Mesulam, 'Essentials of Primary Progressive Aphasia', 17.

[92] Mandana Modirrousta, Bruce H Price, and Bradford C Dickerson, 'Neuropsychiatric Symptoms in Primary Progressive Aphasia: Phenomenology, Pathophysiology, and Approach to Assessment and Treatment', *Neurodegenerative Disease Management*, 3.2 (2013), 133–46 <https://doi.org/10.2217/nmt.13.6>.

[93] 'PPAInformation2016.Pdf'.

[94] Francesca Caso and others, 'In Vivo Signatures of Nonfluent/Agrammatic Primary Progressive Aphasia Caused by FTLD

Pathology', *Neurology*, 82.3 (2014), 239–47 <https://doi.org/10.1212/WNL.0000000000000031>.

[95] 'Primary Progressive Aphasia', *Cleveland Clinic* <https://my.clevelandclinic.org/health/diseases/17387-primary-progressive-aphasia> [accessed 1 May 2019].

[96] Rachel Wynn, 'What Is Primary Progressive Aphasia?', *Gray Matter Therapy*, 2014 <http://graymattertherapy.com/primary-progressive-aphasia/> [accessed 1 May 2019].

[97] 'PPA-0517-0519-What-Is-PPA_WEB-1.Pdf' <https://www.alzheimersresearchuk.org/wp-content/uploads/2017/07/PPA-0517-0519-What-is-PPA_WEB-1.pdf> [accessed 1 May 2019].

[98] 'Alzheimer Europe - Dementia - Other Forms of Dementia - Neurodegenerative Diseases - Fronto-Temporal Degeneration - Primary Progressive Aphasia (PPA)' <https://www.alzheimer-europe.org/Dementia/Other-forms-of-dementia/Neurodegenerative-diseases/Fronto-Temporal-Degeneration/Primary-Progressive-Aphasia-PPA> [accessed 28 April 2019].

[99] Gabriel C Léger and Nancy Johnson, 'A Review on Primary Progressive Aphasia', *Neuropsychiatric Disease and Treatment*, 3.6 (2007), 745–52 <https://www.ncbi.nlm.nih.gov/pmc/articles/PMC2656316/> [accessed 28 April 2019].

[100] 'Primary Progressive Aphasia | Genetic and Rare Diseases Information Center (GARD) – an NCATS Program' <https://rarediseases.info.nih.gov/diseases/8541/primary-progressive-aphasia> [accessed 28 April 2019].

[101] Genetics Home Reference, 'What Is a Gene Mutation and How Do Mutations Occur?', *Genetics Home Reference* <https://ghr.nlm.nih.gov/primer/mutationsanddisorders/genemutation> [accessed 28 April 2019].

[102] Valéria Santoro Bahia, Leonel Tadao Takada, and Vincent Deramecourt, 'Neuropathology of Frontotemporal Lobar Degeneration: A Review', *Dementia & Neuropsychologia*, 7.1 (2013), 19–26 <https://doi.org/10.1590/S1980-57642013DN70100004>.

[103] Michel Goedert and Maria Grazia Spillantini, 'Pathogenesis of the Tauopathies', *Journal of Molecular Neuroscience: MN*, 45.3 (2011), 425–31 <https://doi.org/10.1007/s12031-011-9593-4>.

[104] 'Frontotemporal Dementias' <http://neuropathology-web.org/chapter9/chapter9cFTD.html> [accessed 28 April 2019].

[105] Adam L. Boxer and others, 'Frontotemporal Degeneration, the next Therapeutic Frontier: Molecules and Animal Models for Frontotemporal Degeneration Drug Development', *Alzheimer's & Dementia: The Journal of the Alzheimer's Association*, 9.2 (2013), 176–88 <https://doi.org/10.1016/j.jalz.2012.03.002>.

[106] Manuela Neumann and others, 'Ubiquitinated TDP-43 in Frontotemporal Lobar Degeneration and Amyotrophic Lateral Sclerosis', *Science (New York, N.Y.)*, 314.5796 (2006), 130–33 <https://doi.org/10.1126/science.1134108>.

[107] Rachel H. Tan and others, 'TDP-43 Proteinopathies: Pathological Identification of Brain Regions Differentiating Clinical Phenotypes', *Brain*, 138.10 (2015), 3110–22 <https://doi.org/10.1093/brain/awv220>.

[108] Genetics Home Reference, 'TARDBP Gene', *Genetics Home Reference* <https://ghr.nlm.nih.gov/gene/TARDBP> [accessed 29 April 2019].

[109] Rachel H. Tan and others, 'TDP-43 Proteinopathies: Pathological Identification of Brain Regions Differentiating Clinical Phenotypes', *Brain: A Journal of Neurology*, 138.Pt 10 (2015), 3110–22 <https://doi.org/10.1093/brain/awv220>.

[110] 'Symptoms & Causes of PPA' <https://www.brain.northwestern.edu/dementia/ppa/symptoms-causes.html> [accessed 29 April 2019].

[111] Alon Seifan and others, 'Childhood Learning Disabilities and Atypical Dementia: A Retrospective Chart Review', *PLoS ONE*, 10.6 (2015) <https://doi.org/10.1371/journal.pone.0129919>.

[112] Emily Rogalski and others, 'Increased Frequency of Learning Disability in Patients with Primary Progressive Aphasia and Their First-Degree Relatives', *Archives of Neurology*, 65.2 (2008), 244–48 <https://doi.org/10.1001/archneurol.2007.34>.

[113] Seifan and others.

[114] Zachary A. Miller and others, 'Prevalence of Mathematical and Visuospatial Learning Disabilities in Patients With Posterior Cortical Atrophy', *JAMA Neurology*, 75.6 (2018), 728–37 <https://doi.org/10.1001/jamaneurol.2018.0395>.

[115] Betsy Simmons Hannibal and Attorney, 'How to Write a Living Will', *Www.Nolo.Com* <https://www.nolo.com/legal-encyclopedia/how-write-living-will.html> [accessed 21 November 2019].

[116] 'Power of Attorney' <https://www.americanbar.org/groups/real_property_trust_estate/resources/estate_planning/power_of_attorney/> [accessed 22 November 2019].

[117] 'Treatment and Management of Lewy Body Dementia', *National Institute on Aging* <https://www.nia.nih.gov/health/treatment-and-management-lewy-body-dementia> [accessed 24 April 2019].

Printed in Great Britain
by Amazon